THE 17 HOUR FAST™

Dr. Frank Merritt
and Phil White

To Wu family,

Thanks for being such
great friends. It's been
fun watching Steven & Levi
grow up together.

THE 17 HOUR FAST
Copyright © 2018, Dr. Frank Merritt & Phil White

Vitality Pro, LLC, a research company
dedicated to improving quality of life and athletic performance
through development of innovative modalities, techniques, and systems.

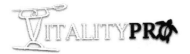

For more information, visit myvitalitypro.com
or email: vitalitydoc@yahoo.com.

This book is written
in memory of my best friend,
Jason Smith.

This book is dedicated to anyone who
has faced failure and initially thought, "I can't,"
then defiantly stood back up and said, "Yes, I can."
My best friend Jason was given only months to live,
but courageously he, his wife, and friends teamed up and said,
"We can beat this." And we did for over 7 years.

If you're battling cancer;
if you have vascular disease such as heart disease or stroke;
if you have high blood pressure, high cholesterol, or type 2 diabetes;
if you struggle with obesity and metabolic syndromes;
if you have depression and/or anxiety;
if you're an athlete aspiring for the next level;
if you suffer from a broken relationship;
you can win.

The 17 Hour Fast is not just about health-related conditions,
it's about choosing to be a victor and not a victim.
This book is dedicated to the champion and challenger alike
because every champion will face defeat and
every challenger has a champion inside.

When you say, "Look at all my failures and/or all the
adversity in front of me," then I say, "Perfect."
Failures and adversity are the secret ingredients for growth.
You just need to know how to properly use them for future success.
This book can help. It is dedicated to YOU!

DISCLAIMER

The 17 Hour Fast is for educational purposes only. This book does not provide medical advice and is not a substitute for professional medical examination or diagnosis and treatment. Consult with your doctor or healthcare provider before beginning any aspect of *The 17 Hour Fast* or any new diet, exercise, or health program. As discussed in this book, moderate intermittent fasting provides health benefits for most people. However, fasting may pose health risks for some participants depending on individual health and fitness. Participation in any fasting including *The 17 Hour Fast* is the sole discretion and responsibility of the participant.

CONTENTS

ACKNOWLEDGMENTS

Thank you to the team of people who helped me work on this book:

- Kim, Kate, and Gabe—for graciously allowing me to share your story and keep my promise to Jason.
- Regina—for your love, encouragement, and assistance with proofreading and editing
- Samuel and Levi—for your love and sacrificing some "daddy time"
- George Merritt—for exemplifying fasting in our home when I was growing up
- Wanda Merritt—for a lifetime of support as a mom
- Phil and Nicole—for your partnership on this book
- Brandon Rager—for the book cover art, website, and workouts
- Peter Furler—for your guidance and surf breaks
- Randy Rarick—for teaching me the true meaning of "aloha"
- Gene Stallings—for your "life lessons" and encouraging me to go to Haiti with "Live Beyond"
- Jeremiah Castille—for your mentorship and powerful prayers of encouragement
- Each of our contributors—for your collective wisdom, talent, and insights: Mac Powell, General Mark McQueen, Barry Zito, Sam George, Brian Mackenzie, Jesse Billauer, and Jack Reece

FRANK MERRITT, MD

• • •

I sign most emails "Gratefully" because it reminds me how thankful I am for so much, to so many. First, thank you to Frank for the privilege of collaborating with and learning from you on this project. My goal with every book is to tell a story that changes lives, and your friendship has certainly changed mine. That gratitude extends to your wife, Regina, and sons Samuel and Levi, for sharing your time with me during this project. I'm profoundly grateful to my other co-author and friend Brian Mackenzie for introducing me to Frank through our book *Unplugged* and making me realize what an impact his work was having. I was privileged to also meet Brandon Rager through that book. He was kind to design the cover for this one and again shared his expertise in the text.

Thanks also to all our featured contributors, including those like my good friend Andy Galpin whose words didn't make it into the final manuscript. Your stories added a lot to the narrative and the lessons you generously shared—like Sam George building a life defined by memories not possessions and Randy Rarick taking time to enjoy simple pleasures—have left an indelible mark on me. I appreciate the ever-present support and encouragement from my parents Veronica and Ian and siblings Barrie, Jacqui, and Debbie, plus Molly, Ollie, Mike, and Lisa Flounders, and Nick Whitfield.

Janice, Dave, and Randall Stephens (and Nicole and Hilde), I will be forever grateful to you for letting me share John's story, which I hope will positively impact everyone who reads it. Then there are the friends who always get behind my writing and indulge me rattling on about the latest book topic, including Brett Chalmers, Henry Worcester, Tom Seibold, Rodger and Kelli Fernandez, Ben Spicer, Jono Lloyd, Justen and Liz Wack, Luke Crisell, Brett Yoho, Jon Manley, Matt Cormier, Craig Babcock, Kenny Kane, Kai "Borg" Garcia, Mike and Jason Slattery, Jordan Olivero, Paul and Jenny Hunt, Chris Frankel, Fergus Connolly, Kevin Kerr, Ian McMahan, Dan Vanderpool, and Pete Hitzeman.

Thank you to my sons Harry and Johnny for being patient with me when Frank and I were on the phone talking fasting yet again. Finally, thank you to my wife and long suffering editor-in-chief Nicole, who transcribed, edited, and much more throughout the course of this project, and is my everything. My contribution to this book is dedicated to my late, great father-in-law, John Stephens.

PHIL WHITE

INTRODUCTION

THE PROMISE

I never wanted to write a book. I'm a doctor, not a writer. I like science and barely got a B in English composition. But I made a promise, one that I cannot and will not break. Not a simple promise, like agreeing not to tell your best friend's secret. This promise is a lifelong commitment. And if I learned anything from growing up in a small town in Alabama, it's that you keep your commitments or die trying.

In September of 2009, my wife and I took our newborn son to meet his "uncle," our dear friend Jason. I remember it well. Jason and I were rocking in the chairs on his front porch. He had spent the past seven years fighting brain cancer. Jason's battle had been a beautiful balance of both courageous fight and graceful acceptance. Now, again, the cancer had come back and was mounting a terrible assault. Jason, who had never before asked me to make a promise, now asked me to promise him one thing. He stopped rocking his chair, looked me straight in the eyes, and asked me to continue the research that we had begun to aid in his battle and to use that research along with his story to save and improve the lives of others. He was serious, so after quick contemplation, I promised. I didn't know it then, but that would be the last time I would see Jason.

JASON'S STORY

In the summer of 2002, Jason and his beautiful wife purchased the house across the street from ours in Dothan, Alabama. Jason had just graduated from law school and was starting his first job as an attorney with a local law firm. We were all about the same age and at the same point in life—just one year earlier, my wife and I had purchased our first home as I began practicing medicine. With similar interests and hobbies, we became instant best friends. A former college athlete, Jason enjoyed a vigorous, athletic lifestyle.

One day, Jason passed out during an intense exercise routine. The subsequent trip to the doctor's office would change their lives forever. The results of a routine MRI were anything but routine. Jason was diagnosed with brain cancer and had only months to live. While he received the best care modern medicine could offer, his wife recruited close family and friends to review research from both traditional and alternative sources on nutrition, fasting, exercise physiology, thermal therapy, recovery, and much more.

Jason changed his lifestyle in accordance with many of these findings. He'd initially been given six months to live; he "lived" for more than seven years. During this time, Jason was a loving husband, fathered two children, savored great relationships with friends, and practiced law. Equally important, through his example Jason taught everyone around him the beauty of life and the importance of love. Jason fulfilled his purpose.

THE JOURNEY

Why do we meet certain people in our lives? Why do we go through hardships, trials, and tribulations? After Jason's death, I wrestled with these questions. During this period, a friend of mine gave me a quote that had given him strength during tough times. It reads, "And not only that, but we also glory in tribulations, knowing that tribulation produces perseverance; and perseverance, character; and character, hope," (Romans 5:3-4 NKJV). Initially, I questioned what hope and happiness could ever come from Jason's death. But I was reading the quote all wrong. It doesn't mean that hope will passively or automatically come to you after the tribulations. On the contrary, it means that you have to actively work through the tribulations with perseverance, and that you must open the door for positive change in your own life and the lives of others. Only then will you have hope.

After Jason's death in 2009, I focused on our growing family and my career in emergency medicine. During this period, I served as both emergency physician and medical director of our trauma center at Bay Medical Sacred Heart and continued my work with many athletes, including NASCAR drivers, professional surfers, Ironman triathletes, and football players and teams, both as a physician and in advanced training innovation.

It was during the Pipeline Masters in Hawaii in December 2014 that I was challenged to keep that promise to Jason. I was providing medical support for the surfers during the event and was staying with the Johnson family. While we were watching the event from the Johnsons' backyard, the conversation turned in a direction that led me to tell Jason's story. With excitement, several in our group asked what I had done to fulfill the promise. I told them that I had shared many of the research findings with many of my patients and athletes. This group then advised me that my promise was worthy of a grander production, such as a foundation or research company. Feeling a little ashamed, I spent the rest of the trip and the next two months pondering what to do with Jason's story and our research. After much prayer, meditation, and discussion with my wife and close friends, I committed to a dedicated research sabbatical starting in May 2015, which meant that I turned in my notice to leave full-time ER practice. Goodbye to all the usual and known, and welcome to the unpredictable and unknown!

We set up our sabbatical home at Pepperdine University, which is where I had conducted research in the early 1990s. There, we reconnected with former friends and professors, including esteemed biology professor Dr. Steve Davis and his wife, Janet. I had remained friends with many members of the Pepperdine faculty and staff, and they were supportive of our sabbatical and helped us in every way possible. As we began the research, friends, athletes, and researchers were eager to participate and assist us.

Most of all, it was wonderful to see firsthand the talent of my wife, Regina, as a physical therapist. Her functional view of human anatomy and physiology led us to understand the need for integrative solutions—this was the breakthrough of the research sabbatical. Anyway, I could go on and on about God's providence and all the wonderful people and friends who gave generously of their time and talents. Truly, it was like Jason was directing the entire sabbatical from heaven.

As the summer drew to an end, my hospital back home contacted me and proposed a contract that would bring me back to my ER practice while still leaving me time for this commitment to research and development. It made sense, so my family and I returned back home and created a company called VitalityPro to continue our work. Since then, we have expanded our research and learned more about how to properly integrate nutrition, thermal therapy, breathing, sleep and recovery, and fasting into our daily routines to maximize overall health and performance and minimize injury and illness. We started health camps with strength and conditioning coach and former football player Brandon Rager, as well as free wellness programs for underserved populations.

We continue to openly share our research with other individuals and organizations in an effort to make people's lives better. To make a long story short, Laird Hamilton introduced me to Brian Mackenzie, who introduced me to writer Phil White. Phil has the talent to offset my B in English composition. Additionally, Phil has his own personal story and motivation for wanting to write this book.

I'm writing this book because I'm keeping my promise to Jason. I'm sharing our fasting protocol because it can truly help you live better and longer. I'm writing because my best friend, Jason, wanted you to have this.

In appreciation,

FRANK MERRITT, MD
June 2017

• • •

JOHN'S STORY

I never got to meet my father-in-law. John Stephens loved to laugh, loved playing golf, and loved spending time with his family most of all. Like Frank, he was the son of a small-town preacher, and like the title character in the John Denver song "Matthew," he grew up in the rural Midwest, where money was scarce but joy was plentiful. John had a natural gift for numbers and put it to good use, becoming a professor and eventually vice president of finance at my alma mater, MidAmerica Nazarene University. From the time I arrived on the small, leafy campus in August 2001, I heard his name mentioned often, whether it was by his many friends among the faculty or by people talking about the scholarship named after him that helped other mathematicians fulfill their promise.

But it wasn't until I met John's daughter and my future wife, Nicole, that I grasped his real impact. Recently I read a magazine interview with a much wiser man than me who advised male readers to marry a girl who cares about her father. That certainly described Nicole, who was soon telling me stories about how her dad would let her stay home from school and then treat her to a Taco Bell burrito, always filled the gas tank in her first car, and, when Nicole went off to college in San Diego, told her mom, Janice, "Well, I guess our life's over!" And when I met family friends, it was always "John did this" or "John used to say that," said with smiles even as they cried recalling the memories.

As I write this 15 years later, I see his image reflected in Nicole's laughter, the numerical wizardry of our 7-year-old son, Harry, and the compassion of my 10-year-old son, whom we named after his grandpa. Anytime we're out in the forest near our Colorado home, we think of how much John loved bringing his young family out here every summer, even the times when the camper got a flat, the rooftop luggage container flew open and scattered clothes all over I-70, or a storm collapsed the awning on their camper. This is what a legacy looks like.

A year before Nicole and I met, John passed away from brain cancer. While I laughed along with his family and friends at the funny stories of when he was healthy, I also teared up at the sad stories about his sickness. The seizures. The memory loss. The falls. A vibrant, talkative, outgoing man laid low by an unstoppable disease. The wife, three kids, and countless friends left to grieve.

Then last year, my own mother was diagnosed with breast cancer. Thankfully, a preventative screening enabled her doctor to catch it early. After surgery and a round of radiation treatment, she made a full recovery. But still, the specter of cancer loomed large over our family again.

Soon after her diagnosis, I got a text from Brian Mackenzie. We were in the middle of writing a book called *Unplugged*. Brian told me that he wanted us to interview his friend Dr. Frank Merritt. After a few minutes of talking to Frank, it became obvious to me that he was doing something completely unique. On the one hand, there was his dedication to saving lives as an ER doctor. And on the other was his vocation at VitalityPro, which combined his medical and research expertise with know-how from nutrition/fasting, exercise physiology, and many other areas to improve people's quality of life and performance through health camps and classes. And at the root of everything he was doing was a promise. Frank was overcome with emotion as he shared with me his commitment to his friend Jason, who had valiantly battled and succumbed to the same kind of cancer Nicole's dad had.

After getting to know Frank while working on *Unplugged* and collaborating on a couple of articles for *The Inertia*, he and I began batting around ideas about how we might share more of VitalityPro's research. Then, out of the blue, my phone rang early one morning. Once I'd shaken off the sleepiness that fellow night-owl writers know all too well, I realized that this was no ordinary call. Frank was proposing that we share the fasting protocol that had benefited Jason and had such great potential for helping others too. And after talking briefly with Nicole, who is the developmental and copy editor for all my books, I said yes without any hesitation. Why? Because we both believe that if we'd known Frank when her dad had gotten sick, we could've prolonged his life. Or maybe, if we'd known how effective *The 17 Hour Fast* system could be before that, he would never have gotten cancer in the first place. "You *have* to write this book," Nicole told me. And so we did.

People talk all the time about their passion projects and say things like, "I'd do it for free." I had always thought that was just a cliché. But more fool I for my cynicism, because here we are as a husband-and-wife writing-and-editing team, pouring ink, sweat, and tears into this book and not caring whether it makes us a dime. When you're an author, you usually wait anxiously for the next royalty statement, hoping that your books have brought in enough money to pay the bills and see you through to the next project. But this time, I honestly don't care about the size of that next royalty check or where this book ends up in the sales rankings. All I want is for it to help one person like John. One person like my mom. One person like you. I want this book to mean something to someone, as it does to me and Nicole and Frank and Regina, and to improve or even save their life. That would be more than enough.

Gratefully,

PHIL WHITE
June 2017

The *FASTING* LOWDOWN

Fasting is one of the hottest topics in health and fitness. Each week sees the release of countless magazine articles, news segments, and podcast episodes touting its benefits. Everyone from pro athletes to celebrities to everyday folks are getting in on the act, leading to the release of several books on the subject. Yet while each of these contains a few useful takeaways, there hasn't been a single volume that looks at fasting through an inter-disciplinary lens, establishes a minimum effective dose, or seeks to create a holistic, life-changing experience with a weekly fast as the conduit.

The 17 Hour Fast is that book.

Inspired by his best friend's battle with cancer and drawing on years of experience as an emergency room physician and his research and VitalityPro protocols developed with iconic athletes, elite college sports programs, and some of the world's most respected nutritionists, behavioral psychologists, endocrinologists, and more, Dr. Merritt has created a unique program that brings fasting to the masses. *The 17 Hour Fast* is founded on a bedrock of cutting-edge scientific research and practical knowledge from experts in multiple disciplines, yet it is presented in an intuitive, highly approachable style. If you're new to fasting, you'll find this book easy to understand, and once you're done, you'll be fully equipped to apply its step-by-step approach. If you're already familiar with other fasting protocols or are even an expert on the topic, we hope you'll still find some new and valid information that can expand your thinking.

Unlike the many books that treat fasting like a traditional training program that requires people to progressively increase the frequency and duration of their fasts, *The 17 Hour Fast* only asks you to take one small step: skipping a single breakfast per week. Research shows that 10 percent of Americans rarely eat breakfast and more than half skip it once a week anyway, though this is in an unhealthy context as part of an over-stressed, over-worked lifestyle leading to binge eating and other unhealthy practices.[1] Once you've achieved this step, we'll guide you on a path to perfecting your fasting routine. In the following pages, you'll learn how such a seemingly small weekly commitment can yield big physical, cognitive, and emotional results. *The 17 Hour Fast* also reveals how fasting itself can be a conduit to a whole-life transformation, including deeper relationships, increased self-knowledge, and reduced stress and anxiety. After reading this book, you'll be able to:

- Perform *The 17 Hour Fast* once a week to help you cut cholesterol, reduce bacterial overgrowth, and lower toxins

- Train your liver, pancreas, adrenals, etc. to be more efficient

- Create a rich, fully engaged experience before, during, and after fasting

- Achieve many of the benefits of a 48-hour fast in less than half the time, while avoiding many of the pitfalls or risks of more extreme fasts

- Overcome food-related psychological and behavioral issues while turning destructive habits into healthy ones

- Improve physical and cognitive performance

- Eliminate sugar dependence

- Rediscover your natural "flex fuel" capacity to power your body and mind with both ketogenesis and gluconeogenesis, rather than just relying on frequent sugar top offs

- Reduce oxidative stress and inflammation[2]

- Achieve more restful and restorative sleep

- Use *The 17 Hour Fast* as a catalyst for a full lifestyle transformation

- Give to others in need through the Calorie and Goodwill Exchange program

- Use fasting to strengthen your work-life balance, improve relationships, and focus on helping yourself and others

- Break free of food advertising mind control

- Overcome the negative routine of habitual and boredom-related eating

- Give your digestive system a break and help overcome issues like IBS, fatty liver disease, acid reflux, and more

DIETARY BIOCHEMISTRY 101

W e'll be talking a lot about fats, carbohydrates, and protein in the course of this book, along with glucose and ketones. Instead of making you read an entire dietary biochemistry text, let's make it as simple and pragmatic as possible. Here we go:

FATS (hopefully good and polyunsaturated) are converted into energy through a process called **KETOGENESIS**, which makes ketones. The body uses ketones as fuel.

CARBOHYDRATES (hopefully good and low glycemic index) are broken down into glucose by digestive enzymes along the course of the digestive tract. The body uses glucose as fuel.

PROTEIN is made up of amino acids. These are used as the "building blocks" of body tissues, including muscle. However, if the body needs energy badly, these amino acids can be converted to glucose through the process called **GLUCONEOGENESIS**. The body uses this glucose as fuel. While 13 amino acids are made into glucose, two are made into ketones, and five can be made into either glucose or ketones. So if protein is used for energy, the majority of protein is made into glucose. Remember that when you drink a protein shake. Are you using it for energy or to build muscle? More on that later.

Turn to the following page to see the amino acid breakdown.

Refer back to it as much as you need while enjoying the rest of the book.

AMINO ACID BREAKDOWN

GLUCOGENIC AMINO ACIDS			
alanine	arginine	asparagine	aspartic acid
cysteine	glutamic acid	glutamine	glycine
histidine	methionine	proline	serine
valine			
AMINO ACIDS THAT ARE BOTH GLUCOGENIC AND KETOGENIC			
phenylalanine	threonine	tryptophan	tyrosine
KETOGENIC AMINO ACIDS			
leucine	lysine		

QUICK RECAP

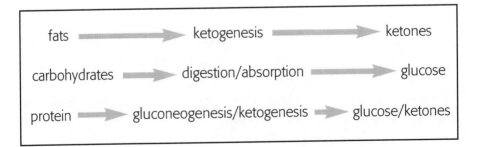

fats ➤ ketogenesis ➤ ketones

carbohydrates ➤ digestion/absorption ➤ glucose

protein ➤ gluconeogenesis/ketogenesis ➤ glucose/ketones

The GREAT FOOD DECEPTION

Before we start addressing our society's dysfunctional relationship with food, its devastating consequences, and how *The 17
Hour Fast* can help, we first need to look back to get a little
perspective on how we got to this point. So let's explore how food's influence
reached super-sized proportions over the past century, what cultural changes
prompted its elevation to an obsession, and the role of advertising, marketing, and branding.

THE MOST MARKETED MEAL
OF THE DAY

When you were a child, how many times did your mom or dad chide you
for skipping breakfast, before going on to remind you that "breakfast is the
most important meal of the day"? In my case, a lot. Same goes with Phil,
despite us growing up 4,000 miles apart—me in Alabama and him in south-
west England. Maybe you say a similar thing to your kids or grandkids. But
have you ever thought about where this saying came from, how it became
pervasive, or, crucially, whether its sentiment is noble or has any evidence-
based science backing it?

We can trace the origin of this ubiquitous phrase back a hundred years.
In 1917, Lenna Cooper wrote an article for *Good Health Magazine* with the
same title as that famous admonition. She suggested that breakfast "should

not be eaten hurriedly, and all the family, so far as possible, should partake of it together. And above all, it should be made up of easily digested foods, and balanced in such a way that the various food elements are present in the right proportions. It should not be a heavy meal, consisting of over five to seven hundred calories."[3]

We can get behind the part about starting your day with your family and not rushing your food. But when we dug a little deeper to get to the real motivation behind Cooper's article, we found something startling. The publisher of *Good Health Magazine* was none other than Dr. John Harvey Kellogg, co-founder of the company that invented flaked cereal back in 1894.[4] When Cooper's article was published, Kellogg and his colleagues were competing with the likes of Postum Cereal Company—whose founder C.W. Post believed that cereal could cure all manner of health problems, including malaria and appendicitis—to make breakfast cereals the morning go-to for millions of Americans. Cooper's story became their manifesto.[5]

We're not villainizing these efforts as we remember that these were different times involving two world wars, the Great Depression, and the Dust Bowl, during which many Americans were undernourished or suffered from malnutrition. For such people, fortified cereals played an important role in their nutrition.

Over the next few decades, the cereal companies upped the ante, not only targeting moms and dads but also creating demand among their children with colorful branding that included characters like the Rice Krispies elves, who made their first whimsical appearance in the 1930s. The following decade saw cereal manufacturers introducing marketing gimmicks like commemorative pins and plastic toys to make their wares even more appealing to kids.[6] And in 1944, General Foods staked their claim to America's breakfast tables by putting "Breakfast is the most important meal of the day" at the center of an ambitious advertising campaign. Supermarket staff handed out thousands of pamphlets explaining why nutritionists believed breakfast was so significant and all the reasons that cereal was the best thing to feed a family first thing in the morning. Meanwhile, General Foods' radio and print ads tied the "most important meal" notion to productivity, proclaiming, "Eat a Good Breakfast—Do a Better Job."[7] Soon enough, America was hooked on cereal and these marketing claims became widely accepted facts.

It wasn't just breakfast that became big business in the early and mid-20th century, but food in general. Before the so-called golden age of advertising depicted in *Mad Men,* food sat in its rightful place as part of a healthy, balanced, and active lifestyle for most people. But as soon as food producers started employing Madison Avenue agencies, our society's relationship to what we eat and drink was forever altered, and not for the better. We soon became convinced that food was synonymous with fun, needed to be consumed quickly via fast food and microwave dinners so we could keep pace in our increasingly frantic world, and should be conveniently packaged instead of carefully cultivated, harvested, and eaten. At the same time as such ideas were taking hold in the 40s, 50s, and 60s, many family farms were bought out by huge agribusiness conglomerates. As a result, we lost our connection to where food comes from, what it takes to grow it, and how to enjoy reasonable portions not tainted by chemicals or other toxins.

Toward the end of the 20th century, how we view food shifted again. With the rise of cable television came multiple channels dedicated to food and chefs who became global celebrities. While fast food ads still touted the benefits of instant food gratification and snack companies reinforced the ties between their products and sports events, we also began to see the other extreme—soft focus, slow motion cinematography that elevated food beyond a merely sensory experience to a sensual one promising something so delicious that it was almost taboo. The next generation of those clever mad men once again made food into more than it should be, not to mention making us believe that we're hungry at all hours of the day and night. Given our country's serious body weight issues, that's the last thing we need!

It's no coincidence that the prevalence of psychological diseases related to food started to skyrocket. At one extreme are the dysmorphic conditions like anorexia and bulimia, whose sufferers struggle with guilt and denial-related issues regarding food. At the other end of the spectrum are those who are driven to excessive consumption, whose challenges are represented in the fact that we now have the highest percentage of overweight and obese people in the history of our country. If you struggle with such challenges, our hearts go out to you and we hope this book can help you start making positive changes in your life.

THE CONSEQUENCES OF MORE

When something in our life isn't fulfilling, we should either cut back on it or change it. And yet what we often decide to do instead is to add more of it: more work so we don't focus on our unsatisfying job; more workouts to try and make this unenjoyable, unproductive exercise routine yield better results; and more activities to crowd out any time for what we fear might be painful self-reflection. This certainly applies to food too. The response to our largely flavorless diet is usually not to start growing our own herbs or to learn how to cook rich dishes with fresh ingredients, but rather to add more sugar, more salt, and more artificial flavors to ever-larger portions.

In addition to the big issue of how much we eat, there's also the consideration of what we're taking in. The average American consumes 160 pounds of refined sugar a year, a full 70 pounds more than in 1900.[8] So what has all this extra sugar wrought? Well for starters, it has compromised the ability of the liver to function as it is supposed to. The liver should be able to fuel our cells through both ketogenesis and gluconeogenesis, but when we take in refined carbs every few hours as if we were hooked up to a sugar IV, it starts favoring carbohydrate digestion/absorption and neglecting fuel production from non-carbohydrate sources. The function of the pancreas and other organs is also disrupted.

Over time, this manifests itself in a broad range of life-threatening conditions. Diabetes, hypertension, and high triglycerides and LDL cholesterol combine to create atherosclerosis, which in layman's terms is plaque buildup in the arteries. The effects of this aren't limited to heart disease alone but also strokes (due to the restriction of blood flow to the brain) and peripheral vascular disease (PVD). These conditions kill the majority of Americans.

We now know that cancer is also tied to high blood sugar levels, obesity, and metabolic syndromes that stem from a distorted relationship with food. In addition, there's a strong causation link between an unhealthy, high-sugar diet and neurocognitive conditions such as ADHD, which often affect children. Other contributing factors include a lack of exercise and artificial food additives. In addition, a 2013 *New England Journal of Medicine* study found a strong association between high blood-glucose levels and degenerative brain diseases like dementia, including Alzheimer's.[9]

There are also diet- and obesity-related diseases that can negatively impact quality of life. Some of these are hormonal, like polycystic ovarian syndrome, which correlates to elevated body mass index (BMI). Men's hormone levels are also adversely affected by obesity, leading to a maelstrom of dreaded conditions (more on that later). Type 2 diabetes brought on by dietary issues is also a cause of men's impotence as the smallest blood vessels are affected. Digestive conditions like fatty liver disease, irritable bowel disease (IBS), and bacterial overgrowth stem in part from poor food choices and chronic overeating. We're also wearing out our bodies much faster than we should because we've created eating schedules built on habitualized hunger, whereby we eat when we're bored, to reward ourselves, and to satisfy societal expectations, rather than eating when we're actually hungry.[10]

Indeed, such reward systems start early. There are many classrooms in which children receive candy or gift cards to fast food restaurants when they excel on a project. (The biggest irony Phil has seen with this was his son getting a McDonald's gift card for hitting a target in PE!) A lot of parents also reward or bribe their kids with food in exchange for good behavior or the absence of misbehavior. At birthday parties and seasonal school celebrations, the treats are primarily sugary, to say nothing of the overindulgence at Easter and Halloween. Then there are the juice box and sports drink breaks in youth sports practices and games. So by the time our children hit adolescence, they're already conditioned to expect some kind of food-related treat (and usually a junk-food one at that) when they do something well and anytime there's a celebration. Years of reinforcement makes it difficult to short circuit this habit and replace it with a healthier reward system.

THE BLESSING OR CURSE OF CHOICE

The greatest gift we have in life is free will. We have the ability to choose, and those choices in large part dictate the course of our lives. Unfortunately, misapplication and misunderstandings regarding molecular and genetic research have led some to believe in what we call genetic fatalism. This genetic fatalism has almost become a presupposition or at least a defining world view—one in which personal responsibility and choices are futile and unable to alter the course of our life beyond our predestined molecular and genetic path. Although we respect the role that our DNA and other molecules play in determining who we are as individuals, we reject the lens of genetic fatalism. First, none of us know the exact degree to which our genetics or personal choices impact our life's path. Once again, we say that our choices dictate the larger portion. But more importantly, from a pragmatic point of view, at this time in history we cannot alter our genetics. But we can alter our choices. Even if and when genetic intervention is available, choice intervention will remain faster, easier, and less expensive.

So again, the greatest gift we have in life is free will. But with all the temptations and opportunities to pursue things that aren't beneficial, it's very easy for our biggest blessing to become our biggest curse. This is certainly the case when it comes to the relationship of Western societies to food. Most of the world is trying to find more calories, but we have ready access—at the supermarket, in our refrigerators and pantries, and in fast food drive-through lines—to far more calories than anyone could ever need or could hope to consume without having health problems. Some can have a perfectly functional relationship with food, but for all too many, the sheer abundance, ease of access, and array of choices is overwhelming and food becomes something it was never intended to be—an overindulgence, a fixation, and the source of behavioral addiction. Then you throw in the mind control of the advertising industry and snack and junk foods that have been fine tuned to create a desire for more and more, and you can suddenly spiral out of control with your eating habits.

This is not to say that we think you're a bad person, weak, or in some way lacking if you are overweight, obese, or struggle with an eating addiction or disorder. Many people in our own families have battled obesity for much of their lives. We believe that, just like them, you are a person of great value, and we want to help you, through this book, to restore your relationship with food and to reframe your body image. It might seem like a small thing to just miss one meal a week. You might be thinking, "Come on, Dr. Merritt, how can that *possibly* work?" But we've seen over and over again that by fasting and creating new habits that we will introduce over the coming pages, people just like you—and in many cases, worse off—have indeed turned their lives around and found the health and balance they had long thought to be impossible. You can do it, and we're privileged to be right here beside you as guides, encouragers, and teammates. Yes, teammates, because we battle this foe together.

If you're a person who is exercising regularly, has a body composition in the "healthy" range, and eats mainly unprocessed, organic, and whole foods, then well done! We are glad you're already making sound choices. But we still believe that while you're not starting from the same position as someone who is sedentary, overweight, and eats poorly, you can still utilize this book and *The 17 Hour Fast* system to find opportunities for further improvement in your life. Maybe you check most of the boxes of a balanced and healthful life but are still hooked on sugar. Perhaps you're very physically fit but struggle to recover and frequently battle injury.

It could be that you have a very successful career but are stressed out to the max and have little time to spend with friends or family. We want to meet you where you are, help you identify areas for growth, and then provide you with a road map to make these advances. If you're an athlete, perhaps you'll be tempted to skip to chapter 10, Fasting for High Performance. While you will find that section beneficial, we urge you to stick with the logical progression of the preceding chapters as you might find some value in them. Or if you simply must skip ahead, please come back and read the rest of the book afterward.

PSYCHOLOGY OF OBESITY AND METABOLIC SYNDROMES

If we're to help you overcome food-related challenges, we can't just look at actions and behaviors, but also the mindset that drives them and the habits and compulsions this creates. Simply put, "As we think, we behave." That's why one of the disciplines we've worked closely with in creating *The 17 Hour Fast* is psychology. Before you can start to reap the physical benefits that fasting can deliver, we first need to help you reframe your attitude, beliefs, and thought processes surrounding food and its place in your daily life.

THE ORIGINS OF THE KETOGENIC DIET

The ketogenic diet has been used historically in medicine to treat epileptics and others suffering from seizures and has also been shown to benefit many other conditions. Even if you're not focused on consuming meals that are high in fat, moderate in protein, and low in carbs, you can use *The 17 Hour Fast* to start getting some of the benefits and reawakening your liver's capability to power your cells with both largely untapped ketogenesis and improved gluconeogenesis. That said, this is not a book about the ketogenic diet. If you want to read one of those, we suggest you start with Jimmy Moore and Eric C. Westman's *Keto Clarity* and Leanne Vogel's *The Keto Diet*.

Have you ever seen one of those food ads where someone cuts into a piece of chocolate cake and that delicious waterfall of sugary goodness oozes down the side of it? That's the kind of sensuality that our culture has attached to food and has made several cable channels must-see TV for a new generation of foodies. Master chefs have become famous and accumulated massive online followings, and we're exposed to hundreds of food ads each day via multiple digital and print mediums. Food is all around us, and because it's so readily accessible, it's all too easy to complete the connection between food ads, our Pavlovian response, and our overindulgence. As a result, far too many of us are dying from diseases of choice.

It might not seem like missing one meal a week could do anything to break this cycle and put food back in its proper place. But we've seen that it can. And it's not just the fasting itself, but some of the associated practices we'll explore in the upcoming chapters, like intentionally cutting yourself off from advertising with an accompanying technology fast, focusing on other people instead, and regaining a sense of perspective by giving to those who don't have enough to eat to survive. We're not saying that food is bad, but our attitude toward it needs to be reframed.

When you have a bad habit, we know that from a behavioral psychology standpoint you can't just get rid of it. Instead, you must replace it with something else, and this needs to provide a reward that gives you the same hit of feel-good neurotransmitters (we could just copy and paste Charles Duhigg's book *The Power of Habit* here, but we don't think Charles would like that, so just go read it).

The 17 Hour Fast can help you in this area by setting up new habits that provide alternative rewards instead of the sugary snacks we like to treat ourselves with. We know plenty of people who've told us that once they started fasting weekly, they stopped snacking out of boredom and were able to break self-destructive eating patterns driven by habit and convention, rather than by actual hunger. Some of them soon realized that those times when they thought they were hungry they were actually thirsty, while others have said that they've stopped rushing through big piles of bland fare and are now savoring smaller portions of higher-quality and better-tasting foods.

MISSING *the* MARK

I n her book *Deep Nutrition,* Catherine Shanahan writes that we've been misled into believing "the notion that if we ever got sick, modern medicine would come to our rescue."[11] As an emergency medicine doctor, I have spent a portion of my career "rescuing" patients from the catastrophic conclusion of their lifestyle choices. Even when we were successful in saving their lives, we could not undo the long-term damage that was irreversible.

Modern medicine is amazing, and over the past 19 years, I have been privileged to work alongside some of the most talented and selfless doctors, nurses, and other healthcare professionals (not to forget equally talented administrators and support staff). I'm also grateful that I get to interface with some of the best technology the world has to offer.

Once again, practicing medicine and "rescuing" others in their hour of need has been my occupational passion. Since making my promise to Jason, my focus has simply shifted to helping them avoid that catastrophic "hour of need" as well as empowering them to enjoy a more fruitful and abundant life.

In fact, medicine has created many "rescue nets." There are bariatric medical doctors who can test for and treat underlying metabolic diseases such as hypothyroidism and furthermore can prescribe medications to aid in weight loss. There are surgeons who are skilled at various bariatric procedures including gastric modifications and liposuction, just to name a couple. Other rescue nets that are often underutilized include behavioral psychologists, nutritionists, and health and fitness experts.

Nonetheless, two thirds of American adults and a third of our children are overweight or obese, leading to $200 billion a year in medical costs from the related heart and metabolic diseases. For all the so-called wonder drugs and technological advances in medical care, we are, as Shanahan rightly points out, "sicker than ever."[12]

This isn't because we don't have smart scientists, well-equipped hospitals, or dedicated doctors and nurses. I know from firsthand experience that we do. It's because we were wrong to believe that we are subject to the whims of destiny and fate, like the doomed hero in a novel or its Hollywood movie adaptation. In order to make our lives better, we need to reclaim primary responsibility for ourselves and the consequences of our actions.

Part of the problem is that we've failed to acknowledge the cause and effect relationship of our behaviors and the debilitating and life-ending diseases that continue to ravage us. This is why we need to change our thinking and recognize that every decision we make with regards to our bodies—to exercise or not, to eat enough or too much, and so on—has profound consequences. When we're at the grocery store, whether we choose to stick to the healthy offerings on the perimeter or the processed foods in the middle aisles matters. Every item you put in your cart moves you closer to life or death. This might sound dramatic, but seeing what I've witnessed in the emergency room day in and day out, I know it's true because I've seen the manifestation of repeated poor choices.

We live in a society that is not just addicted to sugary foods, but also may have an overreliance on pills. We seem to believe that we can behave however we want and make as many bad decisions as we like, because there just has to be a tablet or capsule out there that will undo all the ensuing problems. We've become used to getting food fast, so we reason that the remedy to our overconsumption must be just as quick and easy and will solve our problems.

Then we have fad diets that captivate the imagination of journalists, TV hosts, bloggers, and the audiences they serve for a while, but soon fade away when the next big thing comes along a couple of months later. First we heard that we should be eating a low-fat diet. Then it was a low-sugar diet. Next a high-protein diet was in vogue. Then it was high fat. And round and round we go. Moderation and common sense aren't "cool" and don't generate hype. Marketers also realize that we all have an inner zealot inside us who likes to go all in on something, get with like-minded people as part of an in group, and tell everyone else what they're doing is wrong. So we keep bouncing from one extreme to another, believing that maybe this time we'll find the answer to our health problems, even though experience should tell us that extremism isn't going to work.

As a friend of mine often says, we're living in the Excited States of America, where we go all in for the latest celebrity-endorsed "craze" for a couple of months and then cast it aside when something newer and shinier shows up. Certainly this is true when it comes to how we're told to eat. This can be a geographical thing like the Mediterranean diet or French cooking. Or diets that center on a certain macronutrient-based approach, such as the South Beach diet, the Atkins diet, the Paleo diet, or anything in between (not to say that there's no merit in these, but rather that we blow hot and cold when it comes to how we should eat). It's also the case with exercise, from jogging and aerobics in the '80s to high intensity training in the '90s to home workout programs in the 2000s capturing headlines for a while and then falling out of favor. Yet for all this hype and all these supposed cure-all diet and exercise trends, we have just as many food-related issues as ever and arguably more so.

Another challenging part of this discussion centers on surgical procedures that seek to curb people's overeating. I know some wonderful bariatric surgeons who do fine work and have committed their careers to helping people. Not one of them believes that the procedures they perform are the cure-all for obesity and related metabolic and digestive disorders. This is why they want their patients to enroll in and stick with cognitive and behavioral therapy programs before and after their surgeries—so they can learn to change their thinking and their resulting habits that have gotten them into this state in the first place. It's pointless for someone to have a gastroplasty (aka stomach stapling), liposuction, or some other procedure if they are going to leave the hospital and go right back to their old bad habits. There has to be a willingness to change and the professional support to help facilitate lasting positive alterations in behavior.

WE THINK, THEREFORE WE EAT

What we've got to do is take an axe to the root of our issues with food: our thinking. If we go for physical actions first, we're going to have limited and short-term-only success if we cannot and will not alter our perspective and our mindset.

So what's first when we start to consider how to alter our thinking toward food? We've got to overcome the dominant cultural narrative that we're mere subjects of our destiny and fate. If you look at some popular movies, you'll see this philosophy at work. *Star Wars* is the most successful movie franchise of all time and just one of the many big box-office hits predicated on the idea of fate. TV shows and popular music reinforce this notion that we're just little leaves being twirled around by this big river of life and are helpless to swim against the current.

We also see this storyline play out in the medical community and how we view genetics. How many times have you heard someone explain their obesity or inability to lose weight by saying something like, "I just have bad genes"? Certainly, there are some genetic conditions that mean people put on or find it hard to lose weight, as Sylvia Tara expertly explains in *The Secret Life of Fat.* But these are typically rare. Most of us might be limited to a small degree by our DNA but can still largely influence how our genetics are expressed by the daily nutritional, exercise, and sleep choices we make.

If you're someone who has thrown up your hands and decided that you're a prisoner of fate, we want you to check that mentality now and entertain the notion that maybe you have far more control over your health and your life than you and others have given you credit for. In the ER, I see some of the sickest people in the country, and I have witnessed firsthand that when they start to take back control of their lives and stop giving in to the false doctrine of destiny, they often make a dramatic turnaround and significantly improve their quality of life. You can too, but it has to start with you retaking responsibility for yourself. We believe *The 17 Hour Fast* can show you how strong you really are.

On the surface, this book might seem like it's about skipping one meal a week. But the bigger topic here is choice and how you use the decisions that you make all day long to move you closer to poor health and death or, we hope, to a rich, full, long life. We can help get you started on the positive path, but we need you to be an active partner if you're going to reach your full potential. As silly as it might sound, we want you to go to a mirror right now, look yourself in the eye, and see a champion. Tell that victor who's reflected back at you, "I am in control of my life." Now let's learn a little more about how this champion can change for good with a simple, easy-to-follow fasting protocol.

The 17 HOUR FAST SOLUTION

What if we could hit a big reset button and recalibrate the way we act toward and think about food, rewire our eating habits, and reposition food as something to be savored but not overindulged in or exalted? What if we could improve not only our eating choices, but also reduce our stress levels, set better boundaries in our lifestyle, and make some much-needed room to focus on ourselves amidst the clamor and clatter of daily life? What if we could strengthen not only our bodies, but also our relationships with loved ones and those in need? We can, beginning with *The 17 Hour Fast.*

HEALTH BENEFITS OF *THE 17 HOUR FAST*

This section could really be its own stand-alone title focused on the list of benefits you can derive from doing *The 17 Hour Fast* once a week. But because we want you to actually get to the next chapter and finish this book, we'll try to be as succinct as possible. There's a list of resources at the end of the book so you can read more widely, and if you like research as much as we do, we've included references so that you can dive deeper. For now, we think it would be helpful to break up some of the advantages fasting provides into categories (even though many of them overlap, are multifactorial, and could arguably be put under different headers).

Cardiovascular System

Cardiovascular disease—which includes heart disease and peripheral vascular disease—is the number one cause of death for both men and women in the US. Another atherosclerotic disease, stroke, is the fifth leading cause of death in our country. A lot of books rightly focus on our need to improve the health of our heart and entire cardiovascular system through "cardiovascular exercise." Physical activity is a key component of enhancing our cardiovascular health, but we also cannot discount the massive role that our eating habits play. I've put this subsection first because as an ER doctor, I have the heartbreak of seeing young people who are sick and dying before their time because their cardiovascular system cannot overcome their poor food choices.

There are five major risk factors for cardiovascular disease and stroke: high blood pressure (hypertension), diabetes, elevated bad cholesterol, smoking, and family history of cardiovascular disease. As you cannot change your family history and we do not advise smoking, let's focus on the first three. We believe that *The 17 Hour Fast* can help improve your cardiovascular health through the following benefits:

- *Lowering the chance of developing hypertension/high blood pressure*

A high BMI is one of the biggest factors in creating and perpetuating hypertension and blood pressure-related issues. Imagine running a hose from your outside water faucet to a sprinkler in your yard. If there's just one sprinkler, a low faucet pressure will probably be sufficient to generate good water flow to it. This is like someone who's within the healthy BMI range. But now imagine adding four sprinklers to that same faucet. It would take a higher faucet pressure to generate good water flow to all five sprinklers. This represents someone with an elevated BMI.

The same is true of blood pressure in someone who's too heavy. To ensure each cell in the body is getting the blood perfusion it needs, your body has to dial up blood pressure. Over time, this takes its toll on the vessels and organs, including the heart and brain. Sure, you might use medicines to get your blood pressure down, but this is a treatment and not the solution if obesity is the root cause.

Gradually reducing your weight by fasting can help get to the root of the issue and start to bring your blood pressure back down to a safer level naturally.

With the meals surrounding your fast, we're advising that you cut your portion sizes down, eventually getting to 75 or even 50 percent of your usual calorie intake. If you can start sticking to this at every meal, you will begin to lose excess fat, lower BMI, and, as a direct result, aid in reducing your blood pressure.

- *Decreasing diabetes and insulin resistance*

The more sugar we ingest and the higher our BMI, the more insulin resistant our body becomes, which is one of the mechanisms leading to type 2 diabetes. Additionally, there are many pre-diabetics—those with blood glucose levels just under the diabetic threshold number—who can still cause irreversible damage to their health for 10 to 20 years before progressing into and officially being diagnosed with diabetes.

Fasting can help reset our insulin-related processes, increasing our sensitivity to insulin. We amplify this positive impact through the new eating habits the fast encourages, including less snacking, portion control, and reducing the impact of simple sugars that create complex problems. Taking such steps will also reduce blood glucose levels and help the body exert greater glycemic control. And let's not forget that diabetes usually does not exist in isolation, but is closely correlated to the other cardiovascular disease risk factors of hypertension and high cholesterol along with other metabolic syndromes, which fasting also benefits.

- *Reduce LDL ("bad") cholesterol*

Another of the "big five" risk factors for cardiovascular disease is a high level of LDL or "bad" cholesterol, which can cross damaged endothelium, entering the wall of the arteries. That causes your white blood cells to stream in to digest the LDL, resulting in inflammation. Over time, cholesterol and cells become plaque in the wall of the artery. There are more than $26 billion worth of cholesterol-reducing statins prescribed each year. And this is likely to increase with the introduction of new pharmaceuticals that cost $14,600 per patient annually, which could add an additional $23 billion to total annual spending on cholesterol drugs.[13]

But there's another way to bring down bad cholesterol numbers: start fasting. We've seen people reduce their bad cholesterol just by doing *The 17 Hour Fast* once a week. This has enabled some, with guidance from their doctor, to reduce or eventually taper off their cholesterol medication. Please consult with your doctor before doing so.

Cancer

Cancer is the number two cause of death in the US behind cardiovascular disease. In 1990, 26 percent of people in America smoked. Only 11 percent were considered obese. Now, we've got smoking down to 18 percent, so that's a huge accomplishment. But over the same time period, we've tripled our obesity rate from 11 to 33 percent and that's even with loosening up the criteria for obesity. Do you think that with smoking going down and obesity going up since 1990 to 2015, cancer rates went up or down? Sadly, they went up. This is partly because being overweight is a leading contributor to many cancers. *The 17 Hour Fast* can help in the following ways:

- *Reducing adipose tissue (that'd be fat) to lower the risk of certain cancers*

We know from organizations like Cancer Treatment Centers of America (CTCA) that being overweight increases the risk of developing cancers of the liver, gall bladder, pancreas, esophagus, colon, and many other areas of the body and that being obese increases the incidence even more. In fact, CTCA states that at least one out of every 10 cancer diagnoses can be tied to obesity.[14] We're not going to make the kind of fat loss claims that fad diet pill manufacturers do, but by committing to intentionally missing a meal once a week you can start to lose excess weight and change your body composition. This positive effect will be furthered if you can reduce the percentage of carbs you consume in keeping with our guidelines for the pre- and post-fast meals and the accompanying calorie reduction suggestions. Our hope is that if you're someone who wants or needs to reduce your body fat and weight that you can then stick to reduced portion sizes and a better macronutrient mix. Doing so will encourage safe and sustainable changes that will not only take you out of the obese or overweight categories, but also reduce your cancer risks too.

- *Starving cancer cells of sugar to slow or even stop their growth*

As far back as the 1980s, the director of the Meyer Cancer Center at Weill Cornell Medical College, Dr. Lewis Cantley, found that when the relationship between insulin-like growth factor (IGF-1) and insulin goes haywire, tumor growth that manifests itself as breast, colorectal, and other cancer types gets kick-started. He told Sam Apple of *The New York Times* that "It's cells behaving as though insulin were telling it [the tumor] to take up glucose all the time and grow."[15] Such findings have led to scientists at the cutting edge of treating cancer as a metabolic disease to advocate starving such cancer types by severely restricting sugar intake, which may cut off the glucose they use to continue growing and spreading.[16]

The protocols in this book will not put you into the same kind of ketosis that diets with extreme carb limiting do. But they will at least increase the percentage of ketones that your body is supplying your cells with, while decreasing the amount of glucose produced. In addition, the pre- and post-fast lunches and dinners we recommend are low in carbs, and we also advocate cutting out sugary snacks between meals when you're not fasting, further reducing your sugar consumption.

- *Helping your body stop the spread of cancer cells before tumors grow out of control*

All of us have the potential to produce malignant or "cancer" cells somewhere in our bodies at any given time. If our immune system is functioning optimally, it takes care of these before they start rapidly dividing and cause clinical cancer. But when our eating habits are consistently reckless, we start to disrupt this process and get in our own body's way when it comes to cancer prevention.

The mechanism for this is three-fold. First, as we already touched on, eating too much sugar throws the pancreas's insulin-regulation mechanism out of whack. This sends insulin-like growth factor levels skyrocketing, and in the presence of certain types of cancer cells, this is a recipe for disaster because the mutant cells start perpetuating faster than the immune system can keep up.

Second, studies suggest that when we're obese we start to produce too much of the hormone leptin, which fuels cell proliferation and encourages the cancer to grow even more rapidly. And third, we don't make enough adiponectin, which at the right level inhibits tumor growth.[17] So we see an increase of two substances that are speeding up the spread of mutant cells and a decrease of one that's meant to inhibit cancer—a bad trifecta. By reducing the body weight and high body fat that leads to this perfect storm, *The 17 Hour Fast* can help here as well.

Musculoskeletal and Organ Systems

When someone is overweight, they're putting a lot of wear and tear on themselves. From a musculoskeletal perspective, every pound of body weight you add puts multiple pounds of stress on your joints. This is one of the reasons there are 600,000 knee replacement surgeries in the US each year, not to mention the many prescriptions and physical therapy and other treatment modalities. But while such effects are easier to see because they're external, being too heavy also takes a big toll on the multiple internal organ systems that are less obvious. Think about someone building a one-story house. The HVAC systems they put in are intended to adequately heat and cool it. But say they sell the house and someone adds on a second story. If they don't put in a more powerful furnace and air conditioner, the infrastructure is going to struggle to keep up with the demands of this extra square footage. Eventually, the furnace and air conditioner are going to wear out because they're pulling double duty.

The same goes for the heart, lungs, and other organ systems when we're carrying around too much weight. They have to continually work at high capacity just to keep up with the needs of a bigger body. This is another area where fasting can help. As we begin to condition your body to eat less and less often, you're going to start to shed some of that excess body weight, reducing the toll on your skeletal framework and vital organs.

Digestive System

Our digestive system is being asked to do more than ever before and to do it more often. Habitual overeating is asking our gut to run an ultramarathon day after day. And just as even the most elite endurance athletes would break down under such a load, so too does the digestive system start to show signs of wear and tear. From GERD (acid reflux), dysphagia and IBS symptoms of bloating and gas to more serious conditions, we're seeing an increasing number of people whose overloaded guts are rebelling and effectively saying, "Enough is enough." Think about it. If someone has a digestive condition and is admitted to the hospital, the first order from the doctor is NPO, which means nothing to eat. See the common denominator. Here are some ways *The 17 Hour Fast* can answer the call:

- *Clearing out overgrowth of "bad" bacteria*

We're already spending an awful lot on probiotics, and this is expected to balloon to as much as $64 billion worldwide by 2023.[18] Some of us are trying to improve the diversity of our microbiome and increase production of healthy/good bacteria through the use of pre- and probiotic pills and products with active cultures, such as Greek yogurt, kombucha, and kimchi. Additionally, doctors can prescribe specific antibiotics to eradicate this overgrowth of specific strains of bacteria. This is an effective measure, but once again, can be costly and inconvenient.

During my career, I have had many GI doctor (gastroenterologist) colleagues tell me how therapeutic the process of a "colon or bowel prep" can be for their patients. Even though the EGD or colonoscopy is performed to be primarily diagnostic (to investigate and maybe rule out a certain disease), many patients report improvements in certain symptoms for at least a transient period after the procedure. One current gastroenterologist friend of mine said, "It's simple, first we make them have a reduced select lunch, then start the 'Prep,' which flushes their digestive system out. Then it's only clear fluids and broth for supper, then fasting with only water until the procedure." If you're like me and have had an EGD or colonoscopy, you know this is true and also that you don't eat until after the procedure is finished, sometime between 9 AM and noon. My esteemed friend attributes a large part of the therapeutic effects to a "tapered fast and flush" prior to the procedure.

In this book, you'll discover how tapered fasting can encourage your body to flush out an overgrowth of bacteria and toxins and put your gut microbes back in balance. The recent trend of eating many little meals every two to three hours has replaced the time-tested balance that eating two to three meals a day provided. These "mini-meals" provide the bacteria with a constant source of nutrients to grow and, in this case, overgrow. No longer is there the "fill-up and flush-out" mechanism that two to three meals a day and occasional fasting provided. So just the very act of not eating for a while can offer the chance for some long-overdue weekly housekeeping of the digestive tract.

- *Retraining the pancreas and liver to run on a "flex fuel" blend of ketones and glucose*

In the elite performance world, there's always a lot of chatter about the effects of detraining/deconditioning and the loss in muscle mass, decline in skills, and other issues this can lead to. Yet how many times have you heard anyone suggest that the liver and pancreas can suffer from detraining? We're guessing you answered, "Never."

And yet many of us face this very issue. The pancreas helps regulate our body's energy by the release of insulin, glucagon, and other hormones to direct the liver and other cells. A high-carbohydrate diet leads to the body running primarily on glucose alone. Because there's plenty of glucose available from digestion, the liver doesn't use the mechanisms of gluconeogenesis (glucose production from non-carbohydrates) or ketogenesis as much, and over time, it becomes less efficient at these processes. That means the body is living primarily on glucose from digestion alone. Over time, the liver becomes less efficient at producing slower-acting energy through ketogenesis, which is when the liver produces energy from fats and two amino acids. Our cells also become deconditioned at using this kind of glucose-ketone flex fuel that we get when we eat less carbs and more good fats or when we fast. Weekly fasting helps with this, not only letting the pancreas restore endocrine balance for a while but also encouraging the liver to start becoming better at producing some ketones and our cells to improve how they run off them.

- *Giving the overtaxed digestive system a well-deserved rest*

Almost every system in our body gets a rest at some time. Unless you're attempting a round-the-clock endurance world record, your cardiovascular system, pulmonary system, and musculoskeletal system are going to get a break when you're not training or competing. Your brain gets to chill out a bit when you're asleep, giving your nervous system a bit of down time. And so on.

But the poor digestive system is always on duty. Because many of us eat a huge dinner and then add in a post-dinner snack or two, we're not even giving it a rest when we're sleeping. No wonder some of us toss and turn a lot, wake up feeling bloated in the night, or get gassy first thing in the morning. *The 17 Hour Fast* isn't asking your digestive system to go on strike but rather just to take a night and a morning off each week. As a result, many people who've tried it have reported that the symptoms of acid reflux (GERD), IBS, and other digestive issues have lessened or gone away completely.

- *Eliminating indigestion caused by stress*

When we're continually stressed out, we get stuck in the sympathetic state that tells our body we're under threat. Our adrenal glands secrete adrenaline and noradrenaline (epinephrine and norepinephrine), which raises our core temperature and increases our heart rate and blood pressure, diverting blood flow from the digestive tract to vital organs and muscles to get us ready for "fight or flight." If we live in a chronic sympathetic or "stressed out" state, then diverting blood flow away from the digestive tract means that we're not digesting properly either. This is an underrated contributing factor to some acute and chronic digestive issues.

We've spent the past 15 years working with behavioral psychologists, pulmonologists, and many other specialists to create accompanying methods for helping you to truly relax and exit that sympathetic state. As a result, you'll improve your digestion, providing relief for some of the troublesome symptoms and conditions you might have been dealing with.

- *Stopping hunger cravings before they start*

When we get stuck in a harmful cycle of eating out of habit and boredom, the mechanisms that are meant to tell us when we're full and when we're truly hungry are affected. As a result, we start to feel hungry when the last thing we need is more food. You'd think that as we get heavier, our impulse to eat would be reduced because the body would know that it had more than enough. Actually, our bodies were made with such a feedback system. Adipose (fat) cells produce leptin, which tells the brain that you're full and not to eat. Unfortunately, our habitual eating despite elevated leptin levels leads the brain to "leptin resistance." In fact, the more excess body weight, the higher the leptin levels and the less the brain listens to the hormone shouting, "Stop eating—we're full!" Like your grandpa who can't hear unless you yell, the leptin receptors in the brain have become desensitized or leptin resistant.[19]

The 17 Hour Fast is not a magic bullet by any means, but it can help to tame hunger. When you get to the Pre- and Post-Fast Meals and Ketotic Sleep sections, you'll see how doing a weekly fast can start to improve the regulatory ability of leptin and ghrelin, resensitizing the brain to the former and helping restore the latter to its natural rhythm throughout the day instead of the abnormal patterns we see in people who overeat.[20] These aren't just involved in driving hunger or providing a feeling of fullness. Leptin is involved in balancing energy, mental performance, and fat storage, while ghrelin has an important role to play in metabolism and bone formation.

A study published in *Obesity Reviews* found that a blood ketone level of 0.5 mM was enough to keep hunger pangs at bay, which is achievable with a brief overnight fast.[21]

We've also worked closely with behavioral psychologists to create some alternative reward mechanisms that can replace food-based rewards that encourage overeating and defaulting to sugar-filled snacks. Once you've successfully completed the fast—and we believe that you will!—you will also prove to yourself that you can kick hunger pangs to the curb and start to differentiate between eating out of necessity and eating out of habit. Some of the people who've been doing *The 17 Hour Fast* for a while have said that they never really feel intense hunger pangs anymore—and this includes many folks who admitted they used to snack every hour or two.

Cognitive Function

When thinking about the ill effects of eating too much, we often focus on the physical ramifications. Yet an elevated BMI, along with elevated and labile (fluctuating) blood sugars, can also have a broad range of adverse effects on the brain as well—from reducing our focus, concentration, and memory to causing long-term cell damage and degeneration. Here are some of the ways fasting weekly can mitigate and even start to reverse such issues:

- *Increasing information retention, recall, and clarity of thinking*

Many who do *The 17 Hour Fast* weekly report thinking more clearly when they're fasting, retaining information better, and having faster recall. We like to call this "ketone clarity." Obviously this is very important when I'm having to remember and implement life-saving protocols during my ER shifts. But even if you don't work in a hospital setting, you're going to want to be your best cognitively. And fasting (along with eating less carbs and more good fats and protein when you're not doing your weekly fast) can help.

OK, enough of the anecdotes and onto the science. In an article for *Scientific American*, UCSF neuroscientist Shelly Fan states that ketones give the brain a more consistent energy supply than glucose and suggests that "A ketogenic diet increases the number of mitochondria, so called 'energy factories,' in brain cells."[22] Now this book isn't asking you to follow a purely ketogenic diet, but through the fast and swapping out a lot of your carbs for more fats and proteins, you will start producing more brain-boosting ketones.

There's also evidence that ketone bodies can help protect your brain cells from damage. We talk a lot about buffering physical stress, but the brain also needs to find ways to deal with the effects of this, such as cell oxidation. A study published in the *Journal of Neuroscience Research* states that when we're using additional ketones to fuel the brain, it activates stress proteins that deal with cell oxidation—which can damage brain cells and accelerate age-related decline—and keep all those little mitochondria stable.[23]

Even though we call it "ketone clarity," part of the "clarity" is due to euglycemia, or stable blood glucose. While fasting or just decreasing your high glycemic index carbohydrates, your body maintains more stable blood sugar levels. More labile blood sugars lead to insulin surges and other hormone variations, which can create mental sluggishness, decreased recall, and "gray out."

- *Improving myelination in the brain, which accelerates skill development and speeds mental processing*

In David Epstein's book *The Sports Gene*, he discusses how we improve skills by increasing the amount of myelin associated with certain pathways in the brain—and that experts are essentially creating ultra-fast, fiber-optic-like connections rather than using the dial-up ones they used to access when they were still novices. Research shows us that myelination requires an adequate supply of ketone bodies, which many of us aren't producing enough of due to our high-carb diets.[24] And in some people, the body actually starts catabolizing (eating) myelin to supply more energy to the brain—not good news when you're trying to improve your skill in playing a sport or an instrument, learning a language, or improving your job performance.[25]

By doing *The 17 Hour Fast* at least once a week, you're going to start getting your brain used to running on more of a glucose/ketone blend more efficiently. As a result, you'll have a better supply of the raw materials needed to hardwire the skills you acquire and develop. Other studies show that a diet that's high in good fats also enhances memory and recall. By encouraging you to replace simple sugar calories with those from good fat and protein sources, the pre- and post-fast meals we'll discuss in a little while can also assist with these crucial mind functions.

Physical Performance

If we were to identify the two biggest issues facing athletes, we'd say they were overtraining/under-recovering and poor nutritional habits. We also mistakenly believe that athletic-looking people are healthy because they have six-pack abs and bulging biceps or because of their impressive performances in competition. But having worked with and tested a broad range of high-performing athletes from NASCAR drivers to college and pro football players to big wave surfers, we can tell you that even some of those who look healthy and perform the best are profoundly unhealthy.

One of the main reasons is a dependence on sugar. Since sports drink companies tell us that we need to down bottles of their sugary beverages before, during, and after workouts, we've been conditioned to think that we need sugary drinks, tabs, gels, etc. to fuel and recover from physical activity. As a result, the liver is constantly churning out short-term glucose fuel, while forgetting how to make longer-lasting ketones. We then perpetuate the need to top up on more fast-acting carbohydrates to keep that glucose coming, while neglecting our innate ability to fuel through ketogenesis (i.e., produce ketone bodies from fat and certain amino acids). One of the main pluses of *The 17 Hour Fast* is that it reminds the liver that it was created for both gluconeogenesis *and* ketogenesis to fuel us for long periods of time. Here are some of the benefits when this happens:

- *Enhancing your ability to go harder for longer without needing sugar top offs*

Retraining the body so that it can produce and run on a fuel mixture that's higher in ketones and lower in sugar will allow athletes to improve power output and sustain this for longer periods without needing to rely on the drinks, goos, and gels that we've convinced ourselves we need to fuel performance. The best way we know to do this is to fast at least once a week and to change up our macronutrient intake when we're not, so we're eating less sugary carbs and more healthy fats and protein.

- *Eliminating energy highs and crashes*

One of the things that athletes crave in both competitions and training is consistency. Yet many struggle with feeling and doing great one day and feeling lousy and underperforming the next. A key reason for this is that they've become reliant on frequent sugar top offs and have bought into the fallacy that they need some kind of high-carb pre-workout supplement. When they're not training, they continue to eat something sugary every hour or two, which further exacerbates the energy highs and lows they struggle with during practice and on game day.

By helping to break such eating habits and replace them with better ones, the fasting method you're about to discover can help eliminate such peaks and valleys and deliver more consistent energy throughout the day, including during physical activity. You'll see much more on this in chapter 10.

- *Improving capability and confidence when you haven't eaten for a few hours*

What if you're in a 5K, 10K, or marathon, get to a water station, and there's no sports drink there because the organizers were short on volunteers? It's probably time for you to panic. But it doesn't have to be that way. Once you start fasting weekly and going without food for 17 hours, sometimes while exercising, you're going to learn that such freak-out moments are more psychological than anything, and you will rediscover your body's ability to fuel itself for extended periods of time with ketones—no sugary sports drinks required. This will also be applicable if you're out running errands with your kids, have to deal with a couple of unexpected meetings at work, or don't have time to eat before getting on a flight.

Endocrine System (Hormones)

If you've read much about the adverse effects of a high sugar diet, you're probably all too aware of the impact it has on blood glucose. But did you know that a high carb diet, constant snacking, and overeating at mealtimes also plays havoc with your hormones? We've already touched on what happens to the hunger and satiety hormones ghrelin and leptin, but the impact is also felt across different branches of the nervous system, leading to emotional volatility, inadequate rest and reparation, disruption of thyroid, adrenal, and other glands, and much more. Fortunately, *The 17 Hour Fast* can help the endocrine system in several ways.

- *Resetting hormonal imbalances and taking the load off the adrenal, thyroid, and other glands*

When I succumb to the temptation to take a couple of those mini candy bars that one of my colleagues insists on putting in a jar in the ER, my blood sugar spikes. In addition to causing the pancreas and liver to react, this calls the endocrine (hormone) system into action. A three-gland system, comprised of the hypothalamus, the pituitary gland, and the adrenals, is largely responsible for maintaining the balance of many bodily functions. And the hormones they secrete don't act in isolation but also trigger hormone release from many other glands in the body.

So when our blood sugar is constantly spiking and crashing, our hormones are on a roller coaster ride. This takes its toll on the glands as well because they're having to respond to these continual fluctuations. When you add together a diet high in carbohydrates and chronic physical and/or emotional stress plus a lack of adequate sleep and recovery, it's not surprising that we're seeing more and more people suffering from endocrine (hormone) disorders. We're not saying that all hormone disorders are caused by high-carb diets and obesity, just that diet and body composition play an important role. The good news is that while such conditions can be very serious, many are treatable. By reducing our carbohydrate/sugar intake and restoring a proper BMI, we can do our part to relieve some of the stress on the endocrine system.

Another way the fast can help your hormones is by creating a sense of relaxation during the "Vacation Night" and "Spa Morning" phases. We know that persistently high levels of cortisol disrupt the endocrine system. If you can calm down while you're fasting and then put some of our new self-care practices into action during the rest of the week, we're confident that you can do your part to help recalibrate your hormones.

- *Boosting growth hormone and testosterone levels to aid muscle repair and growth*

Some athletes we know are reluctant to fast because they're worried that it's going to make them lose muscle or negate their recovery from exercise. This is particularly true of "hard gainers" who struggle to increase and maintain their lean mass. Yet research shows us that, in fact, fasting can support muscle gain by boosting growth hormone and testosterone—by up to 2,000 percent in the case of the former.[26] And while athletes might believe that dramatically increasing the amount of calories they eat will promote muscle gain, some studies suggest that overeating actually suppresses the release of growth hormone.[27] So if you start fasting and stop throwing down protein shakes every couple of hours, you might achieve optimal muscle growth and repair.

Plus, by adding in a little physical activity while you're fasting, you're going to drive your demand for nourishment, so when you break your fast, your body is primed to absorb the nutrients in your post-fast lunch and dinner to fuel the kind of recovery you've always wanted.

- *Restoring wake/sleep hormones*

By following the steps that are outlined later in this book, you can restore the timing and balance of hormones such as melatonin, serotonin, cortisol, and others to create a more reparative sleep. This better sleep, especially the recovery stages of it, will further restore other important hormones such as growth hormone and testosterone. All this will help create the recovery and lifestyle that athletes and non-athletes dream of.

Psychological/Emotional Benefits

When we first started using *The 17 Hour Fast*, it was engineered to create mainly physical advantages. Nonphysical benefits were totally unexpected but welcomed. Many people have reported less depression and anxiety, better control of frustration, and higher self-confidence. *The 17 Hour Fast* can help in the following ways:

- *Achieving a sense of control and self-confidence*

Have you ever felt like your eating was controlling you more than you were controlling your eating? How many times have you sheepishly explained away indulging in a tray of cookies with the excuse, "They just looked too good to say no"? Sometimes we can feel that food has power over us and has rendered us powerless to resist it.

Perhaps this is why some of the people who have benefited the most from *The 17 Hour Fast* were those who were initially reluctant to try it, reasoning that there was no way on earth they could go without eating for a whole 17 hours. But once they were able to overcome this self-doubt, they found that it really wasn't all that hard. After all, if you're getting adequate sleep, you're not even conscious for seven, eight, or nine hours. And, assuming you take the advice as we move through each stage of the fast, the rest of the time you'll be spending on self-care, meaningful engagement with friends and family, and serving others. The time will fly by, and you'll hit that 17-hour mark before you know it.

After successfully completing the fast, you'll find a new sense of accomplishment, and then, as you continue to fast once a week, you'll start to see yourself differently—now a strong, confident individual who has asserted mastery over this part of your life. And when you win here, who knows what other things in your life you can start to get under control as well.

- *Taking on and overcoming addictions*

We've had friends who have told us that the self-empowerment that doing a weekly fast has given them has had the additive effect of helping them overcome other compulsions and addictions. Once they have regained a sense of mastery over food, many people feel that they can conquer anything, particularly those who have struggled with overeating and its negative effects for many years. This is not to undermine the fact that many addictions are so strong that people need outside intervention or professional help. But we know a lot people who've used the willpower they develop during the fast to begin acknowledging, tackling, and overcoming addictive behaviors in other areas of their lives.

- *Stabilizing your mood and emotions*

When we're relying on a constant influx of sugar, our mood often follows the blood sugar level resembling the up-and-down path of a roller coaster at an amusement park. One moment we're up at the apex of that big hill and the next we're screaming down a steep slope. This not only leads to emotional lability, but also energy peaks and valleys that take a toll on our days.

Do you have a short fuse and get ticked off at the slightest provocation? Does getting cut off in traffic send you into an expletive-laced tirade? Do you blow up at family members, friends, or colleagues a lot? The root of such frustration and anger might not be an isolated thing or just tied to your life circumstances. Those of us who eat high-carb diets often fail to realize that sugar has an excitation effect at the cellular level, which can lead to a knee-jerk reaction that begins on a far deeper level than at the knee joint itself.

We're not going to claim that *The 17 Hour Fast* is a cure all for such an issue, and in fact you might be "hangry" (that annoyance you feel when you're hungry). But by reducing your sugar intake and the frequency that you spike your blood glucose levels while introducing an energy blend that's slightly higher in ketones, we believe you can start to settle down on a cellular level, which can have a positive additive effect on how you behave.

When I do *The 17 Hour Fast*, it's usually on days when I'm going to be working in the ER. My ability to deal with people who are sick, sometimes fighting for their very life, is directly related to whether I can stay calm and in command of my emotions. I'm sure your emotions play an equally important role in your occupation and life. After years of practicing the fast, I've realized that I get what is called a "ketone calm" when fasting. This enables me to be a better doctor and colleague when I'm working and a better father and husband when I'm at home. We hope you have a similar experience once you start doing the fast.

Relational/Lifestyle Benefits

- *Creating more rhythmic routines that ease stress and help you safeguard your time*

It used to be that life was more orderly. Before the advent of widely distributed electricity, we rose with the sun and went to bed when night fell. Then we were limited to the use of candles and gas lamps. It was only when the popularization of electric light met the Industrial Revolution's urge to work more hours that we started to get out of sync with natural patterns and ourselves. Graham Moore, who won an Oscar for the screenplay of *The Imitation Game,* wrote a book about Nikola Tesla, George Westinghouse, and Thomas Edison with a very apt title, *The Last Days of Night.* Once we had the ability to turn lights on or off whenever we wished, we started to lose that deep connection with the diurnal rhythm of day and night. In recent times, we've started to see the advent of terms like social jet lag to refer to conditions related to this lack of synchronicity.

In addition, we used to set aside more time to honor religious feasts, whether that's Christmas and Easter for Christians, Ramadan for Muslims, or Yom Kippur for Jews. Beyond this, the concept of a weekly Sabbath (Sundays for most Christians, Saturdays for those in Jewish faith traditions) has fallen out of favor, not least because work, along with anywhere and anytime access to the internet and social media, interfere with what's supposed to be a weekly day set apart for restoration. And unless you're a professor who has tenure, the concept of a longer sabbatical lasting several weeks or even a few months isn't likely a possibility. We've also consigned traditions that used to provide a sense of rhythm to people of faith—like pilgrimage and fasting—to the history books.

Farmers probably have more sense of seasonal rhythms than most of us, because they still have certain times of the year to plant and others to harvest. And yet with the widespread use of pesticides, herbicides, and non-traditional growing methods, certain crops are now available and expected to be on the shelves when we go the supermarket year-round (except when they come from organic farms). Simply put, we've lost many of the traditions and calendar-based practices that once gave a sense of order to our world.

While a weekly fast isn't going to take us back to before the Industrial Revolution or return everyone to a day of devout religious observance, it can in some small way reintroduce a cyclic, weekly discipline into our lives. Beyond just not eating one meal a week, the accompanying Vacation Night and Spa Morning also offer the chance to add in other practices, such as a dedicated night of social time for family or friends, time for mindfulness, meditation and reflection, and a more natural sleep-wake cycle that can help your life seem less topsy-turvy and more purposeful.

A good friend who intentionally maintains a sense of rhythm in his daily life is Sam George, legendary former editor of *Surfer Magazine* and a critically acclaimed director, producer, and screenwriter. When we asked him how he achieves balance in life, Sam explained the powerful and formative role that surfing plays:

> "The rhythm of a wave is ephemeral. It's always changing, and you can never ride the same wave twice. When you're out there, you get in tune with that cosmic exchange of energy that has traveled all the way from New Zealand to get to where you're meeting it for that one moment. It makes you remember that the whole natural world is governed by the tide and other ancient patterns, not our attempts to schedule and force every little thing. What would your life look like if you weren't so concerned about the clock and when you had to be here or there? I think that when you fast you're getting away from your normal process and meal times and allowing yourself to just go with whatever comes next. Then you're able to obtain a different perspective."[28]

- *Restoring work-life balance*

We hear a lot about addictions to alcohol, illegal and prescription drugs, and so on these days. Obviously, these are all very harmful and can destroy the lives of individuals and those around them. Yet the destructive addiction of workaholics that affects many of us has gone largely unmentioned. In fact, our society's value system can perpetuate it. Hard work can be positive when we use this drive to achieve our goals and provide for our families. But it can be difficult to know when to draw the line between this and chronic overwork. For several years, I was our hospital's ER medical director in addition to working my share of shifts in the ER. The benefit was a generous salary and the ability to effect positive change at our hospital.

But when I started to run the numbers, I found that people in my position often don't live to the average American's life expectancy age. That was sobering for me, and if you look it up, you may find sobering data for your lifestyle pace too. Anyway, I enjoyed my profession as a doctor and felt blessed to care for others, but I also wanted more time for my wife and kids as well as time to further my promise to my friend Jason. So I made the decision to resign the role and cut back my number of shifts in the ER. My paychecks have definitely shrunk, but what I've gained in return is priceless. We hope *The 17 Hour Fast* can provide a similar level of balance in your life, whether that's between work and your personal life or any other areas that you realize need recalibrating.

- *Slowing down*

Another benefit that fasting can provide is to help improve your ability to change speeds. We're taught from a young age that the faster and harder we go, the more successful in life we'll be. Maybe that's true from a material standpoint, but at what cost to our wellbeing and our relationships? We've gotten really good at rushing around and pushing ourselves to the max but expend very little conscious effort attempting to slow back down again. After walking across America, our friend Jonathon Stalls started a non-profit organization called Walk2Connect, which encourages people to get outside in community and nature through group walks. His philosophy is "Life at three miles an hour." Jonathon says that we've become convinced that zipping down highways at 60, 70, or 80 miles an hour is the best way to travel. But we miss a lot by going so quickly.

Contrast this with the deliberate, meditative pace that walking demands of us and the rich engagement we can get when we move through our environment on foot. We're not telling you to sell your car but rather advising you to embrace a lifestyle-wide downshift as part of your fast. If you do, we believe you'll get to notice and celebrate the kind of unique experiences TNT anchor and leukemia survivor Ernie Johnson calls "blackberry moments" in his book *Unscripted.* This means those sweet times when you bump into a friend, discover a new trail, or take a moment to listen to a burbling stream. We hope this book encourages you to have such rich daily experiences.

OFFERING A HELPING HAND

In a society that's fixated on what people look like on the outside and that exalts skinny models as the ideal of female beauty and ripped action movie stars as the "perfect" man, it's easy for people to feel marginalized when they don't live up to these seemingly unreachable body types. The reality is that a small percent of people look like that or like the pro athletes who we also idolize.

From the time that kids become aware of their own bodies in adolescence, they start to form opinions of what *attractive* and *ugly* mean. Popular media plays a big role in this, as well as advertisements. Anyone who looks a little different or puts on a bit of extra weight can become quickly marginalized and stigmatized. Puberty often creates body-related hangups that manifest themselves in bulimia, anorexia, and other eating disorders in junior high and high school or, at the other end of the scale, boys trying to bulk up with steroids. If left unresolved, these problems merely perpetuate themselves into the college years and beyond. Others who find themselves off the margins of the popular "in" groups often turn to food as an extrinsic comfort or control mechanism, and this quickly becomes a habit that can soon seem unbreakable.

This downward spiral can go on and on, and merely telling people, "You need to eat better and exercise" typically fails to make a lasting impression or lead to meaningful change. The false promises of the dieting industry encourage people to dive headlong into extreme programs that are hard and unpleasant to stick to, often resulting in a lack of adherence and the so-called "rebound effect," whereby a person's weight drops a little but then shoots up to a higher level than it was before when they quit the diet.

The fitness industry also often fails to help the people who need its potential benefits the most. While we celebrate people who drop a lot of weight on TV shows like *The Biggest Loser*, the drill sergeant trainer can beat certain personality types down and make them remember why they hated

56

high school gym class. Or it can be the program itself that is too demanding as it's designed for people who are already avid exercisers but offers little for the sedentary person who needs a more gradual on ramp. If someone is overweight or obese, they might feel uncomfortable and self-conscious in a gym setting, and some trainers may fail to take this and their other psychological needs into account as they train with workouts that would bring some elite athletes to their knees. As a result, many people who make a concerted effort to become more active for a while find only early disappointment and frustration, leading them to abandon exercise and the hope of ever altering their body composition for the better.

These are only a few of the many ways that people can easily feel defeated and beat down. While we were writing this book, a lady came into ER room seven with shortness of breath. The moment I walked into the room I could smell the cigarette smoke on her clothes. Here's a woman who had been in a fight with her nicotine addiction for many years, winning small victories but then backsliding into defeat again. Now she had an illness that all those cigarettes were just making worse. Her lungs hurt, sure, but she was hurting inside for other reasons too.

I asked her, "Are you still smoking?" She lifted her head up and looked at me with a defeated look in her eyes. "I...I've tried...." she began, but couldn't finish her sentence before she burst into tears. Now some people tell you that when you're a doctor, you need to emotionally distance yourself from your patients and not get too involved. But this poor lady's plight just broke my heart. She'd been fighting her urge to smoke for so long that she was just worn out. Maybe her well-intentioned friends and family had been piling on her, constantly saying, "You've gotta quit." They might have thought they were helping, but at a certain point such words are just another burden for someone like this to bear when they're already struggling under the weight of their own doubts, fears, and maybe even self-loathing.

As this poor lady struggled to confess her inability to quit smoking for good, I looked at her and said, "Sweetie, I can see you're beat down. You're sick. I'm not going to do or say anything to make you feel worse. You might not see it right now, but I know there's a champion inside you." Then I took off my stethoscope and laid it on the bed beside her. I said, "See, I'm not a doctor anymore. I'm another person, just like you. I have my own struggles and insecurities. I'm far from perfect. I'm sorry for what you're going through."

This just broke something in her, and she started crying. She got me in this big old hug and just held onto me for a minute, sobbing into my shoulder. That lady didn't need one more person telling her that she was a loser, that she was weak, or that she was a failure. She needed someone to lift her up, to give her a little self-belief and to show her that whether she smoked or not, they cared about her. I just happened to be in the right place to have the blessing of extending that much-needed grace to her. I'm not sure how much good it did in the long run, but for that moment at least, she felt a bit better about herself.

This is just one example of a person who's been beaten down by their struggles, by other people telling them they're a failure because they can't overcome their addiction. I don't just see this in the emergency room. It's all around us. When I take my children to their sports games, I see that kid hanging his head as his mom or dad screams at him over some little mistake that doesn't matter. Maybe you see it in the friend who just can't get a job, no matter how many interviews she's been to or how hard she's tried. People have so much stuff piled on them that they often feel like they're going to collapse beneath the weight of the world.

To offset our struggles, we try to find coping mechanisms that help dull the pain, at least for a few moments. One of the most common is eating. You feel a rush of excitement from the release of "happy hormones" that your brain secretes when you put that first bite of a cookie in your mouth. The next time you eat a cookie, the same thing happens. "Wow, I like this!" the brain says. So now you've got the cue ("I feel depressed") set, the action (eat a cookie) locked and loaded, and the reward (rush of feel-good hormones) reinforced. Suddenly, you have a cookie habit. As that thought process goes down a certain path of the brain, decision making gets faster and faster. That brain path started as a country dirt road, and two months later it's a super highway. So reaching for that sugary treat becomes an almost autonomous reaction to stress or sadness, and every time you let the cycle run its course, you're reinforcing it.

But though it gives you a short-term sense of satisfaction, you can't keep eating cookies or whatever your comfort food of choice might be without consequences. If you continue to top off your fuel tank with sugary foods, the most noticeable external result is putting on a few pounds. Then a few more. If you don't exercise at all or often enough, inactivity outside of work combined with your desk job compounds that weight gain. Just seeing the bathroom scale register a few pounds is only the tip of the proverbial iceberg. You can't see the damage you're doing inside yourself, from the spiking blood sugar level and insulin resistance to the deconditioning of your liver, which becomes inefficient at producing ketones.

So as your body is getting bigger, your internal systems are getting weaker. As a result, you feel famished if you don't eat every couple of hours, your energy levels crash throughout the day, and your emotions may be all over the place. And it all started with that one cookie. Now you feel even worse about yourself because you've put on weight and just can't seem to shake it. Other people start to point fingers and judge you, piling on yet more stress and heartache. This is truly a vicious cycle that millions of people, perhaps yourself included, find themselves stuck in, feeling powerless to do anything about it no matter how hard they try.

Outside of personal struggles, there are a lot of societal conditions that are making us feel more anxious, stressed out, and fearful than ever before. Our extremely polarized political climate, the lack of educational and job opportunities in our inner cities, and the plight of areas like the Rust Belt leave a lot of us feeling hopeless, sad, and lonely. Though social media can offer the opportunity for connection to hundreds of cyber friends, there are many who have few if any genuine, deep, and caring face-to-face friendships that provide the support needed for positive growth. This lack of anything but superficial online interactions leaves some more isolated than ever before. And if someone is struggling to make positive lifestyle changes, it's hard enough to do it in authentic community, let alone if you feel like you're all by yourself.

If this sounds all too familiar, we're truly sorry. But we want you to know that you're not alone, that there are many others facing similar struggles every day, and that we believe in you. By reading this book, you're showing a commitment to being a better you, and we'll be with you every step of the way. You should also know that everyone in *The 17 Hour Fast* community is rooting for you. We're going to come alongside you and do everything we can to help you regain control over your eating habits and the rest of your life. You're a winner, and you're going to prove that to yourself and anyone who has ever doubted you over the next few days and weeks.

A FAST FOR EVERYONE

This is probably just one of many fasting programs you've picked up from a bookstore shelf or have heard people mention. There are some very good ones out there, such as Dr. Jason Fung and Jimmy Moore's *Complete Guide to Fasting,* but others may fall short by only focusing on the fast itself. This is of course important, but from what I've learned and seen in my own life and the lives of my patients, clients, friends, and family, it's only one part of the puzzle. That's why in the coming chapters you'll come to see the fast as part of a relationship-enriching, stress-busting, health-promoting experience.

This isn't a passive, one-way prescription—here, take this pill because I'm a doctor and I know what's best. Instead, it's an active, two-way exchange. If you fully engage and immerse yourself in the step-by-step program you're about to explore, you will have the chance to not only revitalize your health, but also change the way you think and act and the habits you create. And when you do, we don't want the conversation to end there, but rather for you to share what you're learning with us and *The 17 Hour Fast* community so we can all benefit from your personal insights.

This book is also not a manifesto of more. There are so many self-help books, podcasts, and blogs out there telling you that you're not doing enough, whether that's work, exercise, or in many other areas of your life. In contrast, we're going to go through some steps that empower you to do the opposite and encourage you to evaluate what elements you can cut back on or remove entirely. This does apply to food, yes, but also to other parts of your life that might be causing you undue stress and worry because you're taking them to excess. Or maybe you're letting certain things intrude where they have no business being—like technology taking you away from time with family and friends, work intruding on leisure, and the negativity of this world impeding your capacity for joy.

In this case, we're going to try and help you re-establish boundaries that allow you to recalibrate, so that you can reclaim and better protect parts of your existence that have been swallowed up or diminished. As you learn to say "no" to some things, you'll be saying "yes" to more important ones. While we subtract habits that are limiting your quality of life, we're going to add others back in, like true "you time," a better sleep routine, and intentional morning practices that will calmly set you up for daily success.

The goal is to distill the complexity of a multidisciplinary, evidence-based approach into a series of simple steps that anyone can follow and immediately apply. Nothing you're going to read in the ensuing chapters is set in stone. We want you to tweak, modify, and improve on the guidelines we're going to share so that *The 17 Hour Fast* fits you and your unique needs.

FINDING BALANCE

What we're advocating is not zealous or extreme. It's the pursuit of more moderation, restraint, and balance in your eating habits and your lifestyle, so that you can enjoy vitality today, tomorrow, and for many years to come. We know that the accumulation of the little choices can either take away years from our lives or extend our time on this earth and enhance the quality of it. And the great part is that you're at the crossroads—shorter, lower-quality life this way or longer, higher-quality life that way—with us alongside you to help you choose the right road forward.

This book isn't about Dr. Merritt, Phil, or any of the experts whose knowledge you're about to benefit from. It's the stories of people like you who have inspired us to write this book and pass on what we've learned. From my friend Jason to the college and pro athletes we work with to our family and friends and the

PLANNING FOR YOUR FAST

To ensure that your first fast goes smoothly and that you finish it, we implore you to be deliberate and think about which days during the upcoming week are best to start and end your fast on. When we interviewed our friend Jon Micah Sumrall, the musician and lead singer of the group Kutless, he told us, "To be successful I've got to know how something like fasting is going to help me and improve my life. Then I need a plan of attack like an athlete with their race strategy and goals that I set beforehand. I'm more likely to have a positive experience with something like fasting if I also have parameters to guide me."[28]

patients and clients who've all improved their health and increased their vitality through *The 17 Hour Fast,* this book is about *you.*

Our goal is that this book gives you something positive to grab hold of and embrace and will enable you to not only overcome your own struggles, but to pass on what you've learned to bless others. This is a book for you, first and foremost. But then it becomes a book for those around you who you're going to help.

It doesn't matter what you've done up until this point or what challenges you currently face. What we want you to focus on is what happens next. You're not going to wake up tomorrow and find that all your problems have remarkably vanished, but your first successful *17 Hour Fast* will be a meaningful, purposeful, and intentional step to get you further along the path to a more fulfilling life. If you're already successful, fit, and healthy, you'll still find some secrets in these pages that give you a personal and performance boost you never dreamed possible.

The very act of committing to this initial fast and then joining us in repeating it once a week is a sign that you want to better yourself and make meaningful, positive change in your life. You can then build on this and use the fasting as a springboard to daily, weekly, and monthly improvements, some of which you probably can't even imagine right now. I believe that, just like that lady who broke down and cried on my shoulder in ER room seven, you are a champion.

Right now, you might be saying, "Dr. Merritt, I can't do this. I can't go 17 hours without eating. I can't turn my life around." Hold on a moment. Anytime my kids tell me, "Dad, I can't," I remind them of the word they're forgetting to add to the end of that statement: "yet." That's the first transition I want you to make. From "I can't" to "I can't yet." Then we're going to take it one step further and move from "I can't yet" into "I can." We're fully convinced that if you'll keep working through this book with an open mind and take action on the steps we set out, you're going to overcome your health struggles, transform your life, and do what winners do: win. You've already successfully completed the first play by reading this far. Now let's go finish the game.

HEALTH SCREEN *and* COLLABORATIVE MODEL

One of the shortcomings of existing fasting models is that they expect everyone to be at and be able to get to a certain level. Telling everyone that they must advance to a 48-hour or 72-hour fast is like asking every person in a gym—from the pro athletes to the newbies—to follow an Olympic training system. Sure, the pros would do great, but the everyday Joes would collapse on day one and vow never to set foot in a gym again.

Setting unrealistic or even dangerously extreme goals for fasting makes the false assumption that everyone is healthy, well balanced, and able to withstand the shock to their system that a two- or three-day fast introduces. Not so! As we've already discussed, there are millions of people who are struggling with a wide range of digestive, metabolic, and other diseases, many of which stem from or are exacerbated by their faulty relationship with food. If you're one of those people, know that we don't judge you for where you are on your journey and aren't going to ask you to go to lengths that seem impossible. Rather, we want to meet you right where you find yourself and help you, just like I do with the thousands of critically ill patients I treat in the ER each year. If you're skeptical and think that you're beyond reach, we want to tell you that you're not. And if you think that fasting isn't right for you, we want to convince you that it is—or, at least, that *The 17 Hour Fast* is.

It would be risky for you and irresponsible on our part if we asked you to just blindly follow us right into fasting. Instead, we want to ensure that introducing a weekly fast is a safe choice and that you don't have anything in your current state or medical history that would make you or your doctor feel uncomfortable. As a physician, I have a responsibility to stick to the Hippocratic Oath and "first do no harm." Instead, I want to make sure *The 17 Hour Fast* is going to help you. That's why the first step is to go to your primary care physician and get a health screening to make sure you'll be able to start fasting safely. This evaluation will produce a lot of useful information regarding your health, some for the purposes of this book and additionally other information that your physician and you can use to enhance your overall health.

One thing you do need to pay attention to and discuss with your doctor is your blood glucose (blood sugar) level. Because fasting naturally lowers blood sugar, if you're on medication that is designed to lower blood sugar, you'll need to collaborate with your doctor to tailor your medication plan so you can fast. However, if you have type 1 diabetes, it may not be best to try fasting in general, unless your physician feels differently and can adjust your insulin dosage to allow you to proceed. But, you can still benefit from much of the other valuable information in this book even if you don't fast.

If you have a metabolic condition, high blood pressure, high cholesterol, or any other medical issue, don't let your conversation with your doctor end once you get your test results. We want you to keep the dialogue going so that they can help monitor your progress and the state of your condition. In many cases, the benefits of weekly fasting can help your body normalize, leading your doctor to adjust your medications and overall treatment plan. The body takes time to react, and just like you wouldn't do one workout and expect to break a world record the next day, neither should you expect overnight results. But if you successfully complete this initial fast and then repeat it weekly, continuing to hone your experience as you go, we're convinced that you will start to see noticeable and lasting health benefits. Now let's look at exactly what tests you should be getting and how the results impact what comes next.

HEALTH SCREEN: HOW TO

CAVEAT: This chapter may seem unnecessary to those who are established with a physician. Unfortunately, studies show us that there is a large population of folks in the 20-to-50 age range who feel fine but have silent diseases like high blood pressure and diabetes. One of the goals of this chapter is to capture this population in this screening.

BENEFITS OF SCREENING

At this point, we bet you're raring to go. You'd probably like to go into your doctor's office, have them run some quick test, tell you, "Sure, you can fast," and send you on your way. We understand and embrace your excitement as it's the same attitude we have toward such things. But hold on a moment. First, we would like you to spend a couple of minutes exploring why we're advocating a health screen and how it's going to help you.

Our goal is the same as yours here: that you get a clean bill of health and the green light from your doctor so you can get going with *The 17 Hour Fast* and start seeing the positive growth it can lead to. If that's the case, then we celebrate with you.

But what if you get this screen and it uncovers a health issue, maybe one that prevents you from doing your first fast right away? The natural reaction is to feel downcast or upset, and that's a

THE 17 HOUR FAST—AN INTRODUCTION FOR DOCTORS

If you're a doctor who's reading this, you might be deeply skeptical about fasting or be inquisitive about it. Either way, we understand where you're coming from. We want you to know that while there are some anecdotal pieces of advice and things that might not be strict evidence-based science in these pages, the central concepts are based on research as well as input from experts in many medical and scientific disciplines. Our goal for your patients is the same as yours: to improve their health and quality of life and to do so thoughtfully, moderately, and safely. We hope that you too will benefit from this book and will be encouraged to go away knowing more about fasting. Thank you for keeping an open mind, for your daily dedication, and for making sound decisions on behalf of your patients and their families. We trust that you will be a responsible guide for anyone considering *The 17 Hour Fast* and are grateful for your collaboration, cooperation, and wisdom.

perfectly understandable reaction. If any of the tests or screens in this chapter show something that you initially view as negative, try not to fall into the trap of blowing it all out of proportion. Make an effort to look for the good in the situation and be grateful to your doctor for identifying something that needed to be addressed.

It could be that the condition isn't all that serious and can be either corrected or managed fairly easily. This screening may find something that is easily dealt with now but might have become a much bigger problem later if left undetected and untreated. That scaly rough patch on your back that you've been worrying about for a while might turn out to be pre-cancerous. OK, we said the "C" word, but if caught early on, the dermatologist may be able to freeze it off. However, if you wait two years, it might develop into full-fledged skin cancer, requiring surgery, aggressive radiation, and other forms of unpleasant treatment. This perspective of health screening is very personal to me as my mother had breast cancer. Thankfully she went in for a scheduled checkup, caught it early, and is celebrating her 25th year of being cancer free. It was the same with Phil's mom. In such cases, the old adage "an ounce of prevention is worth a pound of cure" is true when it comes to preventative screening. Too often we think of screens as inconvenient and sometimes unpleasant, but we can't overstate the significance of catching disease early.

My fellow doctors and I often try to explain to our patients, "Early in disease: hard to diagnose, easy to treat. Late in disease: easy to diagnose, hard to treat." Consider these tests to be a worthwhile pre-emptive strike that will help identify any issue early so it can be dealt with immediately and remedied before it progresses into something far worse. This is an opportunity you should seize with both hands. And if something does come up in the test results, we urge you to confront it head on, accept it, and commit to decisive, positive action. In the ER, I have diagnosed too many young women in their 20s and 30s who come in suffering from advanced stages of cervical cancer, as well as men with progressive prostate cancer. If they'd only taken the time to get the available screenings, they could have detected their conditions far sooner before they progressed.

At VitalityPro, we've worked with several world-class athletes who discovered they had high blood pressure despite their elite cardiovascular fitness level. They acted responsibly by starting blood pressure medication, and then they resumed their training, because they recognized that they couldn't just run, bike, or swim the medical condition away. We want you to apply the same mindset to any issue that these tests reveal, whether you're an athlete or not. As you progress through this book, you'll see that a natural remedy to every potential problem is considered first. Weekly fasting and other lifestyle changes can make a big difference over time. But as a medical doctor, I also believe in the power of appropriate medication. If the screening turns up something that requires you to take a pill once a day, then so be it if it allows you to live a healthier and higher quality life.

We don't want you to get the tests recommended in the following section just for your physician to say, "Yes, you can fast" or "No, you shouldn't fast and here's why." The scope of this book goes beyond the fast to your overall health, so we want to make sure that you're doing alright. We want you to form a tighter, more productive relationship with your doctor, which can only be beneficial to you and your family in the long run. Don't wait until something breaks to see the expert. Do scheduled maintenance and prevention just like you would do for your car. Your body deserves even better, and so does your doctor. If they feel like you are taking your health seriously and are trying to be proactive, they're more likely to buy in to what we're discussing in this chapter and invest the time and effort needed to be an enthusiastic partner with you.

PICKING THE RIGHT PHYSICIAN

We're hoping that you already have a good doctor who you and your family have been going to see for years. If that's the case, then great, go ahead and skip to the Time to Get Tested section. If you don't have such a patient-doctor relationship, you need to initiate one. Don't assume that because you're young, you're automatically healthy. While it's true that certain conditions, like dementia, osteoporosis, and macular degeneration are more prevalent among older folks, this doesn't mean that those in their 20s, 30s, and 40s are invulnerable. Nor does it mean that if you're a skilled and clever young professional, like a pilot, architect, or engineer, that you can learn everything you need to know about your health on Wikipedia or WebMD. And don't worry, we will not try to build a bridge after watching a "how to" YouTube video, thinking that suddenly we're qualified structural engineers.

You might be highly qualified in your area or even the best in the world, but medicine isn't your forte. So if you're in this lower age range, discard that faulty notion and your youthful feeling of invincibility. Go start a relationship with a good doctor because it will not only ensure that you can fast safely in the short term, but it will also improve your vitality now and as you get older. Plus, on many insurance plans, you get a free checkup and screen every year or six months. Some insurance companies and corporate wellness plans even incentivize you to get these checkups. So what are you waiting for?

One benefit to this technological age we find ourselves in is transparency. We don't have to rely on a static listing like the Yellow Pages to give us little more than a name, address, and phone number anymore. While we don't believe we can or should base a doctor's worth on an online rating as you might a restaurant on Yelp, a hotel on Trip Advisor, or a toaster on Amazon, you can at least check that your prospective physician is board certified, went to a good medical school, and has the required credentials to meet your needs.

Going a bit further, it's also important that you and your doctor connect on certain things. If you're athletic, you might want to find a physician who embraces an athletic lifestyle as well. Should you be a person of faith, it might be a priority to connect with a doctor who shares your beliefs. Remember that we're not just focusing on the physical. You want someone who will have a holistic outlook that encompasses your mind, body, and spirit.

TIME TO GET TESTED

Now that we've looked at why you should get a health screen and how to find the right physician to partner with, let's move on to the tests and panels themselves.

Complete History and Physical

Many underestimate the value of a good old-fashioned doctor's visit where the doctor first sits down and listens to you. Then after listening to you, he or she focuses in by asking related questions that sharpen the diagnosis. In this day of great technological advances, many are ready to rush to the tests. Whereas these have added much value to the field of medicine, we should not undermine the foundation of medical practice, which is the history and physical.

This visit should include a meaningful discussion about your:

- Past medical history
- Past surgical history
- Current medications, herbals, and supplements
- Allergies
- Family history
- Social history such as drinking, smoking, or drug use and occupational and recreational activities

Later, we provide a list of information you should write down in preparation for your visit. We encourage you to always keep a current concise version of this information on you in case of an emergency.

1. Height, weight, and body mass index (BMI)

While these might seem rudimentary, body weight and composition (relative to your height) are two of the biggest indicators for most of the major illnesses that plague our nation. So get these checked first, and we'll compare your initial numbers to those that your doctor records after you've been doing *The 17 Hour Fast.*

2. Vital signs

Standard vital signs include: resting blood pressure, resting heart rate, resting respiration rate, and oxygen saturations. They are called "vital" because they are a representation of the vital organs that keep us alive. They are also vital to doctors because these few measurements can tell us a lot about a patient's condition.

3. Complete blood count

The complete blood count (CBC) is the best option for a preventative blood screen. If any of these numbers are out of the normal range, this could indicate an infection, anemia, an autoimmune disorder, or a number of other conditions. Your doctor can interpret these results.

4. Chemistry panel

This measures blood levels of electrolytes like sodium, potassium, and calcium, which regulate hundreds of processes in your body. Another advantage of the chemistry 14 panel is that it reveals your kidney/renal function by measuring creatinine and the blood urea nitrogen (BUN) levels. In addition, this panel provides an overview of your liver function.

The chemistry panel also measures your current blood sugar level. This is important, but since you're supposed to be fasting since midnight on the day of your lab testing, this blood sugar level may not be a true indication of your normal daily non-fasting blood sugars.

5. Hemoglobin A1C (HA1C)

Someone smart figured out that a form of glucose attaches to and leaves a layer on red blood cells, and they can measure that layer and tell you your hemoglobin A1C level to get a snapshot of your blood glucose levels over the past three months. That gives us a much more accurate picture of your average daily blood sugars. When you commit to doing *The 17 Hour Fast* once a week, this is one of the biomarkers that could significantly improve when you retest in 6 to 12 months.

6. Lipid panel

This test measures the cholesterol in your blood: LDL ("bad"), HDL ("good"), and total cholesterol as well as triglycerides—fats circulating in your bloodstream. People who commit to *The 17 Hour Fast* can see a reduction in LDL, total cholesterol, and triglycerides after about six months. Plan to fast the day you get blood drawn for this test.

7. Hormone panel

Another thing you might want to get tested is the level of hormones like estrogen and testosterone. Some men truly suffer from low testosterone and should seek expert medical consultation. Later in this book you'll discover some natural ways to boost levels of testosterone and growth hormone.

Menopause and hormone-related disorders such as polycystic ovarian syndrome are sensitive subjects for those affected. That's a discussion for you to have with your obstetrician/gynecologist (OB/GYN doctor). Your OB/GYN can discuss the risks and benefits of hormone replacement and help you individualize your decision.

8. Thyroid or TSH

We want to make sure you don't have hyperthyroidism (overactive) or hypothyroidism (underactive), which can be serious thyroid-related conditions. Thyroid studies are also their own screening test for any bariatric (obese) patient, as hypothyroidism can lead to obesity.

9. Preventative screenings

We just went through a whole list of reasons to get preventative screens done and some hard-hitting examples that we hope convinced you of their importance. Since everyone has different health conditions, family histories, and risk factors, we'll leave it to your doctor to be the judge of which screens are appropriate for you and at what age. Here are some important screens: annual history and physical, Pap smear, mammogram, bone density test, prostate screen, colonoscopy, EKG, chest x-ray, cardiac stress test, and pulmonary function test.

Once again, consult with your physician to see which screens are appropriate for you, as well as any additional screening recommendations.

10. Cardiac and pulmonary screening

Two basic tests I'd like to see patients have as they get older are an EKG and a chest x-ray. Now if these come back negative, I bet you'll be tempted to say, "Well that was a big waste of money." For you sports fans out there, ESPN's Lee Corso would say, "Not so fast." Remember where I work. If you come into the ER complaining of chest pain and related symptoms, the ER doctor will be able to look into your medical record and make a past-to-present comparison, allowing the medical team to provide a more accurate diagnosis and treatment.

If you have a family history of heart disease along with other risk factors, your doctor may recommend a graded exercise test (GXT). You'll be asked to run on a treadmill for just 15 minutes. If you cannot run, then your physician can recommend the modified GXT, which does not require running.

Likewise, if you have risk factors for asthma or COPD, such as a history of smoking, your physician may recommend pulmonary function testing (PFT).

Once again, this non-exhaustive discussion of possible tests and screenings is only meant to stimulate your thinking and encourage your relationship with a primary care physician. You and your doctor can make the final decisions for what is appropriate for you. Then once you're cleared, you can join us in fasting.

11. VitalityPro assessment

This one is only valid if you'd like to come to a VitalityPro Health Camp or live near someone who is certified in our program. Hopefully in the future it will be online for anyone to use. The VitalityPro Health Age screen assesses your health in multiple areas, including cardiovascular and pulmonary health, mobility, muscle fitness, and body composition, and gives you age-matched scores between 20 and 80—with 20 being the youngest possible measurement and 80 the oldest. We then aggregate these scores to give you an overall vitality age. The age-matched scores make it easy to understand if you're prematurely aging. The categorical scores allow clients to know and address their own weaknesses. Everybody has individual strengths and weaknesses, allowing clients to individualize their health initiatives according to their scores. When I first went through our screening process, I scored 22 on cardiovascular and 39 on pulmonary. Appropriately, I was tested for asthma and medically cleared. I then started training with our Pulm-Max pulmonary conditioning program. Later, I retested and managed to get that number down into the 20s. You can learn more at www.myvitalitypro.com.

12. Dermatology screening

If you enjoy outdoor activities and fitness, then we must address skin. First off, let us advise safe sun-exposure hints, such as choosing outdoor activities during non-peak sunlight times. Morning and evening are better. In addition, wear protective products made with sunlight protection, such as SPF, including hats, shirts, lotion, and blocks for starters.

Next, even if you do all the former, schedule that annual dermatology screening. This screening appointment will serve to hopefully catch any problems early when they're usually easier to treat. It also provides the dermatologist with a great opportunity to update you regarding new products and advice.

ATHLETES AREN'T OFF THE HOOK!

If you're an athlete, I'm glad you haven't skipped right to chapter 10. Thanks for sticking with us and waiting to get there in due course. But while we're thankful you're still working through the sections of the book in sequence, we'd also like to give you a word of caution at this point. It's all too easy to say, "I'm an athlete, my health is perfect, and there's no way I need to get all these tests." Having been around pro surfers, football players, and high performers of many kinds during my career, I've heard such a sentiment verbalized hundreds of times. People think that because they can run fast, jump high, and lift heavy weights that they're some kind of superhero who's completely invulnerable.

Newsflash: they're not. Even the greatest athletes of all time have struggled with illness and injury. Michael Jordan missed almost an entire season with a foot injury early in his career. Women's 100-meter world-record holder Florence Griffith-Joyner died from a cardiac event. Bo Jackson saw his two-sport greatness cut short by a persistent hip problem. Others, most notably Lou Gehrig, have battled chronic conditions, while many more deal with illnesses that impact them daily, such as asthma and diabetes. You also see news stories of people who seemed to be in perfect health dropping dead during a marathon or other race maybe because they never got tested for a condition that might have been manageable if it had been detected, but it ended up claiming their life.

So that you don't become a statistic, we urge you to put your achievements and ego to one side for a moment and submit to getting the basic physical and tests/screens we've recommended here. Yes, it might cost you a few hundred bucks and a morning or two, but think about how much money you invest in coaching and gear and how much time you spend training. Consider how it can help you avoid that upcoming injury or illness, therefore helping you set that new personal record. For a comparatively small investment, either you will get peace of mind, knowing that you are indeed healthy, or you will discover something that is most likely treatable if you do something about it now. Don't let your pride get in the way of making the sensible decision here. Get the tests done, and whatever they show, deal with the results with the same commitment you show to your sport every day.

TAPERING OR GOING OFF MEDICATIONS?

This is another topic that we need to proceed cautiously with. Some proponents of fasting become so gung-ho about it that they start to be like those snake-oil salesmen who advertised cure-all elixirs back in Victorian times.

We're not going to stand here and tell you that fasting once a week is going to solve all your health issues, make you bulletproof, and allow you to go off any or all of the medications you may be taking today.

First off, let me say that as a physician, I see two extremes in our culture today regarding prescription medicines. There is one end of the spectrum where people believe medicines can cure all sickness, thus placing too much emphasis on pharmaceuticals and too little on personal habits such as diet, exercise, sleep, etc. On the other end of the spectrum, I've seen people who are wary of doctors and pharmaceutical companies and so refuse the appropriate use of prescription medicines and other therapeutics.

What we must adopt is a balanced and objective approach. We're thankful for pharmaceutical and other medical-related companies and organizations for all their research and development. Realistically, each of us knows of friends or family members whose lives have been saved or whose quality of life improved due to these measures.

Likewise, the medical text chapters regarding diseases such as high blood pressure and cholesterol (along with type 2 diabetes) all start treatment sections with recommendations of "lifestyle modification." This means improving diet, exercise, etc., as mentioned above. Once again, the medical books recommend this first, but some people may need pharmaceuticals in addition or as an initial "bridge" as they start their "lifestyle modification" and wait for the effects. As Laird Hamilton coined it in a discussion we had in 2015, we need "hybrid medicine." Such an approach allows each of us a balanced pursuit of premium health.

That said, we have seen that many people using *The 17 Hour Fast* have been able to taper their medications and, in some cases, either reduce the number of different pharmaceuticals they're taking or even go off their medicine altogether. For example, there's evidence that shows fasting can lead to a double-digit reduction in LDL cholesterol, which is why some people we've worked with who have been on cholesterol medication for years have been able to cut their dose or, eventually, stop taking it. We've seen similar improvements in people's blood pressure, which we believe is not just due to weight reduction and fasting itself but also the beneficial relaxation and restoration outlined in the Vacation Night and Spa Morning chapters coming up. In addition, we've heard countless people say how much *The 17 Hour Fast* has helped with their digestive complaints, from GERD (commonly called acid reflux) to IBS and beyond. This is partly because they're giving their digestive system a periodic rest and their body is taking care of bad bacteria overgrowth and undigested food that may have exacerbated their symptoms over the years.

While we hope that a weekly fast helps you in similar ways (and maybe some others that we haven't yet seen), realize that the body adapts best to gradual change—and that's the way we're going to approach fasting. As we're only going to be altering a few variables a little bit, it is going to take time to see the kind of results that we know you're hungry for (pardon the pun!). You wouldn't walk into a weight room and expect to come out an hour later with LeBron James's leaping ability or JJ Watt's strength, would you? Neither should you expect your first fast to deliver miraculous results. But just as exercise does create some immediate physiological changes, so too will the fast start having positive effects on day one. Remember, physiological studies indicate that it takes approximately three weeks to see the full benefit of what you do today. You just need to be patient and, as with any successful training program, stick with the fast and integrate it into an overall healthy lifestyle in order to realize its full benefits and your full potential.

Before you start making any changes to your medication, please talk to your physician. If he or she sees positive differences in your metrics after you've been fasting weekly for twelve weeks, your doctor may want to start gradually modifying your medications. (Another good reason to get those tests done before you start fasting!)

We need you to be patient and to continue the same spirit of collaboration and cooperation as you've shown throughout this testing/screening process. In addition to letting your physician run the numbers, don't be afraid to share with them how you feel after you've been fasting regularly for a few weeks. Increasing your self-awareness is a big part of the personal adaptation we believe you're going to undergo as a result of doing *The 17 Hour Fast* each week. So how you feel is just as important as what the data indicates, and you should share this with your doctor so they can get a better sense of how you're benefiting from the fasting and the lifestyle changes it initiates.

The following is important information you need to note prior to your doctor visit:

NOT CLEARED FOR *THE 17 HOUR FAST?*

We want to include as many people as possible in this process, but there are those whose age or condition may preclude them from fasting safely. So rather than returning this book, we encourage you to keep reading and try to apply some of the other concepts, including those from the Vacation Night, Spa Morning, and Pre- and Post-Fast Meals chapters. We hope you find them helpful. And as some health conditions are temporary, you may be able to start the fast sometime in the future. Again, we recommend that you talk with your doctor first.

- *Past medical history*

Write down any conditions that you've had in the past or are currently dealing with and, if possible, the dates that they started and ended.

- *Past surgical history*

List any surgical procedures that you've had in the past and the estimated date (even if it's just the year or how old you were at the time) alongside it.

- *Medications, herbals, and supplements*

List every medication you're currently taking, along with the dosage. It would also be beneficial for you to list supplements you're taking or have taken.

- *Allergies*

List all allergies or adverse reactions you have to pharmaceuticals and non-pharmaceuticals alike. Include everything: medicines, food, bee stings, etc.

- *Family history*

Include all medical conditions that anyone in your family (blood related) has or had. Examples include heart disease, diabetes, and cancer (and what type for the latter). Not every condition is influenced by heredity. Your doctor will know which are and which aren't and what preventative measures you should be taking to reduce your odds.

- *Social history*

Include your marital status, occupation, and leisure and recreational activities. It's also important for your physician to know if you drink alcohol, smoke, or use recreational drugs.

In addition to giving a copy of this information to your doctor and asking him or her to add notes as needed, please carry such important information with you in your wallet. If you come into the ER after an accident and are unconscious, knowing what you're allergic to, what medicines you're taking, and your medical and surgical history can literally be a life saver. If your smart phone has a health app, it's also a good idea to enter this information here. If not, you can put it in the notes app that even older phones have.

YOUR METRICS

This chart should include your weight, BMI, body fat percentage, cholesterol, resting blood pressure, resting heart rate, and fasting blood sugar. When you get all of these retested after doing *The 17 Hour Fast* weekly for 6 to 12 months, record the new values in the second row.

	TEST 1 DATE	TEST 2 DATE
weight		
BMI		
body fat percentage		
cholesterol		
resting blood pressure		
resting heart rate		
fasting blood sugar		

PRE-FAST MEALS

Once you've had your health screen, received the results, and obtained the go-ahead from your doctor, you're ready to move on to the first real stage of *The 17 Hour Fast*: pre-fast meals. We've read several books that don't pay any attention to what happens before someone begins a fast. This would be like a jockey taking his horse out to compete in the Kentucky Derby (sorry, I'm from the South and couldn't resist the analogy) without first putting in the necessary prep work at the warm-up track. In order for your fasting experience to be positive and beneficial, you need intentional, tried, and tested methods to bookend it. Start well, finish well, and what's in the middle will largely take care of itself.

This is why we want you to start thinking two meals in advance of your fast. Unless you're a super early riser or a night owl, we advise you to start your fast at 7 PM. So the second-to-last meal you'll enjoy will be lunch. The temptation before starting a fast is to stuff ourselves silly as if we're a bear preparing to hibernate for a long winter. Because we're so used to hits of refined carbs that only provide quick surges of energy and then the inevitable crashes that follow, we've conditioned ourselves physiologically and psychologically to eat every couple of hours. Every time we notice even a hint of hunger, we head to the refrigerator or the pantry. So why do things differently before a fast?

The first thing to recognize is that during the fast, you won't be relying on glucose from your diet to fuel your organs, brain, muscles, and every cell in your body. Rather, you will stop taking in food and your liver (with a little direction from your pancreas) will begin burning non-carbohydrate sources to produce fuel in the form of glucose and ketones. We only have enough carbs in our bodies to keep us going for a couple of hours. But there are about 3,500 calories in just a pound of body fat, so once we become accustomed to burning fat, there's plenty of fuel available on our own bodies to keep us going around the clock.

Despite what some blogs or books might suggest, your body won't suddenly become "fat adapted" and begin only running off ketones. Rather, the fast will help you change your fuel blend a bit, slightly decreasing the amount of glucose and increasing the percentage of ketones. That's why we call it a "flex fuel" concept. Although initially the change will be slight, even a minor adjustment of the fuel blend can have a significant impact on your energy levels and your hunger and, as a result, your eating habits. This in turn will have an additional positive effect that helps you lose excess weight, as well as improve physical and cognitive performance and recovery.

The difference between fueling with glucose and fueling with ketones is like using varying types of wood in a fireplace to achieve different results. My father-in-law Pete loves a real log fire and enjoys cutting down and splitting his own firewood. Some kinds of wood are more combustible, easy to ignite, and make a big fire. But they burn out quickly too. Other types of wood are less combustible and harder to ignite. Yet these give you a consistent fire that lasts a long time. So Pete uses a blend with more of the former to start the fire and then incorporates more of the latter to consistently heat the house throughout the night. Glucose is like that highly combustible wood, while ketones are the slow-burning logs.

So when you're preparing for your first *17 Hour Fast,* we want your metabolism to get used to the fact that it's no longer going to be depending on you throwing a new highly combustible log into its fire every hour or two. To do this, we'd like *both* your pre-fast meals—the lunch you'll eat sometime between noon and 2 PM and the dinner/supper you'll have between 6 PM and 7 PM—to be lower in carbs and higher in healthy fats (polyunsaturated like those in nuts and olive oil), with a little protein thrown in for good measure.

BREAKING DOWN PRE-FAST LUNCH AND DINNER*

The ideal breakdown for your pre-fast meals should be something like what you see below. But make sure you're only changing one variable each time you fast (such as calorie intake vs. macronutrient breakdown). Also recognize that small, sustainable changes are better than going straight from a huge lunch and dinner to a tiny one or from super-high-carb meals to those with very few carbs. A dramatic alteration in either scenario will make you feel awful and start your fast off badly (see more tips for perfecting your fast in chapter 11). That said, here are the macronutrient and calorie percentages to aim for:

PRE-FAST LUNCH

Fat: 35 percent   *Protein:* 35 percent   *Carbs:* 30 percent
Calories: 75 percent of usual lunch. If you're trying to lose weight/bad BMI,
you might taper down to an end goal of 50 percent.

PRE-FAST DINNER

Fat: 40 percent   *Protein:* 40 percent   *Carbs:* 20 percent
Calories: 75 percent of usual dinner initially, and later, as you "perfect" the fast,
you'll taper down to an end goal of 50 percent if you're aiming to lose weight/reduce BMI.

We're going to be realists rather than idealists here and recognize that if you're someone who typically gets 60, 70, or even 80 percent of your calories from carbs, you're going to balk at what you just read. In that case, try to cut your usual carb percentage in half or a gradual 10 percent reduction for each weekly fast for this pre-fast lunch and dinner. We're not aiming for absolute perfection on the first try because as with mastering any skill in life, that's just unrealistic. Another reason we don't want you to change more than one variable at a time with your approach to food is because if you start shaking everything up at once, you won't be able to isolate which change made the positive difference. After you've achieved some success in this first fast, you can then go back and tweak your approach a bit, which we'll cover in more depth in chapter 11. Regardless, you don't have to start weighing your food or do precise macronutrient breakdowns. Remember, the fasting process isn't meant to be yet another stressor in your life, so don't go down the data geek road unless you enjoy crunching numbers. Just take a guess about how the fat, protein, and carb percentages break down, and that'll be fine for now.

* Note: If you're an athlete who struggles to maintain your "fighting weight" or is trying to put on muscle, this breakdown and the one you'll find in the Post-Fast Meals chapter isn't for you. Please see chapter 10 for your protocols.

IDEAL FATS AND PROTEINS FOR PRE-FAST MEALS

Here are some sources of good proteins and fats to include in your pre- and post-fast meals:

- *Avocados*
- *Coconut*
- *Poultry*
- *Beef (lean)*
- *Fish*
- *Cheese, milk, cottage cheese, and other dairy products*
- *Nuts*
- *Seeds*
- *Beans*

PRACTICING PORTION CONTROL

In addition to thinking about *what* we're eating, we also need to think about *how much* we're eating. With physical activity, most injuries occur when we see people trying to make a huge change in their routine. Either they go from being sedentary to going nuts and working out twice a day or a more experienced athlete jumps headlong into a radically different, pro-level routine that's far beyond what they can handle. The body adapts best if we carefully add a couple of pounds to a lift per session or try to shave a few tenths of a second off our best running time. That way, we're introducing just enough of a stimulus to promote change but not overloading our system.

We see similar problems with crash diets that promise to help you lose 30 pounds in 30 days. Is it possible to achieve this kind of radical weight loss so quickly? Certainly, but it's also profoundly unhealthy and some of that will be muscle and water weight. As the body is trying to adapt, there will sometimes be a rebound effect that sees the person who lost a lot of weight in just a few weeks put most of it back on. Such setbacks, which are also common when following fast weight-gain programs and trendy but dangerous workout plans, merely encourage people to go back to making their old lifestyle mistakes. It would be much more prudent to set a realistic and sustainable goal of losing a couple of pounds a week over the course of a few months, and this will allow your body to adjust gradually as its composition changes and you alter your eating and exercise habits.

We should take a similarly cautious and long-term view with this fast. There will be some immediate benefits, but many others—including improvements in liver and pancreas function, promotion of good gut bacteria, and reduction in LDL and total cholesterol—will take months to fully manifest themselves. This isn't a fad or crash plan with flashy numbers and gaudy marketing claims. Rather it's one that seeks continual evolution and has benefits backed by science. So we need to be patient and start gradually, trying to avoid the "I want it now" mentality that can shock the body with massive changes and make you feel wretched. If you go from eating two gigantic meals to eating nothing for 17 hours, you've created a huge difference and are setting yourself up for a discouraging failure. Should you stuff yourself during your pre-fast lunch and dinner and then go from thousands of calories to zero, it would be like cutting the cables attached to an elevator in a New York skyscraper, resulting in it plummeting from the 87th floor all the way to the basement (thanks for the inspiration, John McClane in *Die Hard*).

That's why we encourage you to take your usual lunch and dinner portions and reduce them to 75 percent for these two pre-fast meals. That way, the difference between your final meals and the zero food during the subsequent 17 hours will be a lot smaller, so your body is less likely to freak out and talk you into breaking the fast early. Making small, incremental changes in your pre-fast meals will also help you avoid the mood swings that some people experience while fasting—your family and friends will thank you!

We don't want to get you into a bait-and-switch situation, so we'll be upfront and reveal that the portion reduction we recommend for your pre-fast lunch and dinner will be mirrored in the post-fast meals phase as well. Again, this is not just a fasting book, but one that aims to help you make meaningful, transformative, and long-lasting change in many areas of your life. One of these, as we went over in the first couple of chapters, is reframing your relationship with food. That's why in the pre- and post-fast meal stages, we recommend that you reduce your portions steadily until you're at half of what you'd normally eat (if you're an athlete or other kind of high performer, this might not be the case— see chapter 10 for a more focused protocol that's right for you).

If you're fine with your BMI the way it is, then you can revert back to your normal portions the evening after the fast is over. But if you're trying to lose some weight, get that BMI number down, and improve your body composition so you have less fat and more lean tissue, we challenge you to

SETTING YOU UP FOR GOOD SLEEP

When it comes to exactly what recipes to make and meals to eat in this first stage of the fast, we'd like you to take charge and experiment a bit. To meet the recommended macronutrient breakdowns for your pre-fast lunch and dinner, check out the sidebar of good fats and proteins and add in some low-glycemic carbs from this chart published by University Health News:

www.universityhealthnews.com/daily/nutrition/glycemic-index-chart

When it comes to the latter, we also encourage you to consider incorporating some foods that are rich in tryptophan. This amino acid is a precursor for serotonin (one of the "happy" hormones) and melatonin (the "sleepy" hormone). It's also a precursor for niacin, a B vitamin that is involved in many bodily processes, including energy metabolism, as well as being used in medicine to help lower cholesterol. To enable tryptophan to cross the blood-brain barrier (BBB), we need a few complex carbs, which is where some of those at the lower end of the glycemic index come into play for your pre-fast supper. The following are some of the best natural sources of tryptophan:

Turkey*	Almonds	Cranberries	Pumpkin, sunflower, and chia seeds
Red meat*	Cheese*	Oats	Crabs and shellfish*
Lamb*	Pork*	Beans	Eggs*
Lentils	Fish*	Chicken*	Tofu

* Opt for grass-fed, organic meat and dairy and organic, free-range eggs. Choose wild-caught fish that's low in mercury and other heavy metals when possible.

stick with these smaller meals. You'll be amazed at how quickly your body will change your hunger and appetite baselines if you dedicate yourself to doing *The 17 Hour Fast* just once a week and apply the pre- and post-fast meal guidelines to the rest of your meals throughout the week. We've seen many, many people meet their weight loss, BMI change, and fat reduction goals this way. We believe you can do the same.

TALKING TACTICS

Just as in sports, the military, or the business world, we've got to look at the fast and its goals strategically, and then, as Phil's co-author in *Game Changer*, Fergus Connolly, writes, "Work backward from the game." The primary aim, of course, is for you to complete the fast without giving into the temptation of sneaking a snack. But we don't want you to have to grind your way through like it's an arduous slog!

That's why we've set up some fun and pleasant experiences in the Vacation Night and Spa Morning chapters and have poured 15 years of research into the micro-calculations that form the basis of *The 17 Hour Fast* protocols. As our friends in the armed forces are fond of saying, the advice in these pages are helping to remove randomness and "control the controllables" that can either put us on a path to win or block our way and trip us up. We're also paving the way for you to create a can-do attitude, reinforce some of your good habits, and change some of those that need work. We hope you finish the fast feeling so good that you not only want to do it again next week but also can't wait to tell your family and friends about it as well. To get to this point, you need to set yourself up to succeed (and conversely, not to fail). A big part of this is your mindset and attitude. But what you do with your pre-fast meals—both in terms of composition and quantity—is also going to go a large way to determining the outcome.

Think about a runner who has trained for a marathon or, if they're really gung ho, an ultra-marathon. If they begin those 26.2, 50, or 100 miles like Usain Bolt blasting from the starting blocks in the Olympic 100-meter final, they're going to fall apart very quickly and be unable to meet their goal of finishing the race, let alone achieve any of their time-based aims or podium dreams. They know the pace they need to start with in order to sustain their effort level throughout the entire race and cross that finish line with a smile on their face (well, at least to cross it, hopefully with a grin). And in fact, many racers start off a lot more tentatively than they're capable of and use a negative split strategy, whereby they speed up every mile until they hit a Mo Farah-like sprint finish at the very end of the course.

Having run (or should I say "survived") several marathons and half marathons, I know that race strategy isn't just about pace. You also need to consider your sleep, tapering down your training, weather conditions, course elevation, hydration, and nutrition. Coaches help their athletes put tactics into place for all of these elements and many more.

That's how we're approaching *The 17 Hour Fast*. This isn't some arbitrary scheme that we pulled out of thin air, and just like the race for the marathon runner, the fast doesn't exist in isolation but in the midst of your life. That's why we also have tactics and strategies to set you up for success, which have been created with the help of experts in many specialties of medicine and science as well as in nutrition, psychology, etc. The pre- and post-fast meals are a vital part of this plan. If you can discipline your eating habits going into and coming out of the fast, you'll be much more likely to have a good experience while you're actually fasting.

At our VitalityPro camps, we don't just have pro and college athletes show up. There are members of our armed forces, firefighters, policemen and women, businesspeople, moms and dads, and everything in between. As part of the packet we send out to people before they get here, we ask them not to eat anything after 7 PM and give them the same guidelines as you'll find in this chapter and the Post-Fast Meals section on what to eat and how much before and after their fast. Then they show up and we do some hard work in and out of the pool and ocean for a few hours during their camp morning (our variation of the Spa Morning). From the elite athletes to the stay-at-home parents, not one of them has come to me or our head trainer, Brandon, and said that they had a bad experience in any way. While you certainly can exercise, and we're going to give you some advice in a later chapter, we're "lowering the bar" to raise your chances of winning this first fast. Priority number one at this stage of the fast is to eat less than usual and follow the nutritional breakdown advice as best you can.

Note: If you're a night owl who will be extending the next phase of the fast—the Vacation Night—until midnight or 1 AM, we suggest that you time shift your pre-fast meals. It's probably best to eat your pre-fast lunch between 2 PM and 4 PM and your supper between 8 PM and 10 PM. That way, the hunger pangs that can show up in the first few hours won't hit before you go to bed. If you do shift the fast this way, you'll also need to adjust the end time so you can complete the full 17 hours.

At the other end of the scale, if you're a super early riser, either by nature or necessity, you might want to shift your fast back an hour or two. So maybe you'd eat your first pre-fast meal between 10 AM and noon, your second between 4 PM and 6 PM, and go to bed at 7 PM or 8 PM. You end the fast earlier so you stick with the 17 hours as well. Again, none of this is set in stone. Tinker with the timing so it best suits your personal physiology and lifestyle, and be sure to let us know what works for you on our social media pages.

START HACKING YOUR HORMONES

In a couple of chapters' time, we're going to take a close look at the importance of sleep to getting the most out of *The 17 Hour Fast*. But it's also worth noting that your sleep the night before you begin the fast is significant. Studies suggest that if you get less than six hours of sleep, you may increase insulin resistance, affecting your ability to properly process carbs for up to 72 hours. A lack of sleep or interrupted slumber may also limit your ability to digest fats and protein. One of the ways that we can increase the benefits of the fast to those of a longer one, like a 24- or 36-hour fast, is to begin and end it in a deliberate way that includes adequate rest, low stress, and good nutrition. But to take advantage of this, make sure you get 6 to 8 hours of ZZZs the night before you start.

Another way you can begin the process of balancing out your hormones and other body chemicals is through the pre-fast meals themselves. Enjoying a fresh, all-natural meal with friends or family will also make your brain pump out feel-good neurochemicals that will help you go into the remainder of your evening in a positive mood. If you can ease your way into the fast from a stress perspective, you'll limit your body's production of stress hormones like cortisol. So although we technically say the Vacation Night begins after your pre-fast dinner, it will be even better if you can prep your mind and body during this meal.

We'll get into the sleep-affecting nature of caffeine and alcohol more in the next chapter, but as it also applies in this first stage of *The 17 Hour Fast*, we'd like to say a few words about it here as well. If you usually keep the coffee buzz going into the afternoon and evening, try to have your last cup a couple of hours earlier than usual and/or taper down. Caffeine not only revs you up but can prevent good quality rest too. And if you like an evening alcoholic drink, we suggest you have it with your pre-fast dinner and stick to one glass (or half of your normal consumption) if you can.

THE SLOW FOOD MOVEMENT WAS RIGHT

In the mid-1980s, we saw a group emerge that dubbed itself the "slow food movement." These folks looked at some of the cultures in which meals are prepared painstakingly for hours with family members and friends using fresh, natural ingredients and then savored over a couple of hours. This was a kind of cultural backlash to the speed fast food offers. We can all take a page out of the slow food cookbook. Yes, we can attach too much importance to what we eat, so it becomes something it was not meant to be. But in our microwave, drive-through culture, it's also all too easy to go the other way and let the joy of cooking and sitting down to share a meal with family and friends be lost to the tyranny of busyness.

I vividly remember taking a trip to Mexico to help with a building project in an impoverished village. At the end of a hard day of physical labor, 18 or 20 of us sat around as our hosts prepared a chicken soup. There was less meat in that soup than you'd find in a typical restaurant portion, yet we enjoyed each bite. As we ate, the kids ran around kicking an old soccer ball while we swapped stories and laughed with their parents and grandparents. They had very few material possessions, yet every evening they celebrated as a tight-knit community, were grateful for getting through another day, and welcomed in strangers like us as if we were long-lost relatives.

That's why in this pre-fast meal stage of *The 17 Hour Fast,* we encourage you to get everyone in your house into the kitchen and prepare your pre-fast supper together. Have someone chop vegetables, while somebody else stirs the broth or fetches ingredients from the fridge and pantry. You could take turns each week choosing in advance what you're going to eat that night. Or if your fast is going to be more of a friend-focused affair, ask everyone to bring a dish that they've prepared themselves (and call them out if you spot a supermarket label on a container!). You will all value your meal more if everyone had a hand in preparing it.

Our friend and mentor Randy Rarick, who cofounded the modern professional surfing tour in the 1970s, has more demands on his time than most people, with sponsors, surfers, fellow event organizers, and more clamoring for his attention. Yet he has established and continues to protect a nighttime ritual with his wife before and during dinner. "At around 5 PM, my wife starts preparing dinner," Randy told me. "She's Italian and is a wonderful cook. Our routine is to each have a glass of wine together. Her email address starts with 'surf widow,' and she has to put up with me being gone a lot, so this is our chance to reconnect and make time for each other. We also try to take trips that have nothing to do with surfing, whether that's going to the mountains or to Europe to take in some culture."[29]

Try to recreate Randy's intentional approach to preparing your pre-fast supper. Once you get to the actual eating part, we have two words for you: *slow down*. We get into this pattern where everything is rushed, including how we eat. Like a hyper-efficient assembly line, we've taken it upon ourselves to relentlessly fill each hour, minute, and second with doing things. If we find a pocket of time that's going unused, we shove something else in there because we've been conditioned to believe that this is what productivity looks like. This can have the effect of crowding out the kind of rich life you deserve.

We challenge you to use the fast as an opportunity to look at your life and see where you can do the opposite and create more gaps. And the first one should be for this pre-fast meal. Resolve in advance to shut your work down half an hour earlier. Say no to that social event you've been dreading for weeks. Now divert this time to a relaxing pre-fast supper with the people you care about most. Don't just make space on the front end, but also clear your calendar for the whole evening after this meal, so you can continue the spirit of tranquility into your Vacation Night, which we'll cover in depth in the next chapter.

When it comes to rushing our food, this doesn't just create stress and prevent us from enjoying a nice meal, but it also has physical effects. This country is plagued with issues like GERD, aka acid reflux. This is partly due to our diet, but the fast-forward pace we adopt at the dinner table is also one of the culprits. This is why *The 17 Hour Fast* not only reduces reflux symptoms by helping fine tune what you eat and how often you eat it, but also by encouraging you to sit down and take your time with eating.

We also contend that one of the reasons that we have so many digestive complaints is because there's all this semi- and un-digested food sitting in our bowels. One possible cause is that we don't take time to chew our food, which we sometimes forget is the first step of the digestive process.

Try a quick self-test. Grab a snack, and on the first bite, write down how many times you chew your food before you swallow it. Try to act like you normally would, not like you're trying to change your ways and set a new chewing world record. Now the first time you do the fast, try to increase the number of chews for each bite of your pre-fast meal. We bet you're going to enjoy that lovingly prepared meal all the more.

Chewing more will also enable you to get twice the enjoyment from your pre-fast meals, post-fast meals, and every meal from now on. What are you going to do with that chewing time? Check your email or send a few texts? No! Be present and enjoy what you're eating, as well as the company of those around you. Try to pay attention to the temperature and texture of your food. If it's crisp lettuce from the refrigerator, notice the nice chill on those leaves. If soup is on the menu, appreciate the warmth of each spoonful as it goes down your throat. Next, turn your attention to flavor. If you took the time to follow a recipe made with fresh herbs, vegetables, and good quality meat or cheese, you've probably put together a pretty flavorful meal.

When was the last time you paid attention to the spiciness of curry, the sweetness of a cherry tomato, or the freshness of cilantro? Try to see how many different flavors you can identify in the meal, and ask others what exactly they're tasting. This reminds us of the animated movie *Ratatouille*. You don't need to be a gourmand to appreciate such nuances. But you're only going to notice them if you stop rushing your food and make a conscious effort to appreciate the sensory experience of your pre-fast meal. This doesn't just have to be true for home cooking. Maybe you decide to take your family out to a favorite restaurant or treat a friend to a meal out someplace. You can still tame the tempo of your eating to the point where you can better appreciate each element of what's served up.

Whether you're at home, at a friend's house, or out to eat, consider having your pre-fast dinner outside if weather allows—on a deck, at a park picnic table, on a restaurant patio. It doesn't matter. A lot of the countries we admire when it comes to certain ways of eating take their meals outside, such as France, Spain, and Italy. If you visit those countries, you'll see that Parisians don't want to be stuck indoors with their croissants but would rather sit around a café's outdoor table.

It's the same in the piazzas of Italy, where the stereotypical image of some old guys sitting around with their espressos and newspapers still holds true.

NOT ALL CARBS ARE CREATED EQUAL

When we gave you the macronutrient breakdown for carbs, protein, and fat, it was intended to be a basic, 101-level guideline. But as you start to tweak the fast, you need to realize that some foods are better than others for you in general and for your pre- and post-fast meals. We recommend that you avoid junk and fast food, candy, sweets, and sugary drinks—basically anything with a lot of refined, simple sugars. Eating a salad chock full of different types of lettuce, carrots, cherry tomatoes, and so on is going to be a lot better for you than a candy bar or a can of soda. We also often forget that even things that have been marketed to us as "healthy" often contain a ton of sugar. That's why Regina and I prefer to eat fresh citrus fruit from our own or nearby local trees than drink glasses of juice. If we do put a little juice in our smoothies, we split a few ounces and it's plenty to add just a little sweetness without sending our blood sugar soaring.

For the carbs in your pre-fast lunch and dinner and your post-fast meals, go heavy on vegetables, which will also hydrate you, and include some fruit and whole grains like brown rice, pasta, sprouted bread, oats, or quinoa to hit your carb quota. But even within these categories, veggies, fruits, and grains all contain varying levels of sugar per serving. Some contain fast-digesting fructose and sucrose, while others have what we call resistant starch that takes longer to digest and doesn't spike your blood sugar as much. Here's a table that will clue you in on the glycemic index values for various options:

www.universityhealthnews.com/daily/nutrition/glycemic-index-chart

Many of the homes have nice little outdoor courtyards in the middle of the house, as a focal point. While we might not have the same architectural advantages in America, outdoor furniture is one of the best buys you can make in terms of improving your quality of life. If you have the opportunity to be outdoors, take a cue from these cultures and go al fresco with your pre-fast meals and as many other meals as you can.

DINNER WITH THE STALLINGS

Coach Gene Stallings was a defensive coordinator on Paul "Bear" Bryant's staff for two national championship victories in the 1960s and then returned to the University of Alabama as head coach after stints at Texas A&M and in the NFL to lead the Crimson Tide to a national title and an undefeated season in 1992. We often have an image of coaches toiling around the clock, but this wasn't the case in the Stallings household, even at the pinnacle of his Hall of Fame career. "Every night we had dinner together at the house and sat down around the table," Coach Stallings said. "Sometimes it was 7 PM, other times 8 or 9. I'd go into work early but in the evenings that was the time for me to be with the children and Ruth Ann. If I had some work to do, it had to wait until after my kids were in bed because dinnertime was when we'd all talk and laugh together. It was a special time."[30]

If Coach Stallings could set aside time to eat dinner with his family while leading a team to a national championship, all of us can follow suit. We want you to commit to making this pre-fast meal and the Vacation Night that follows into the same kind of "special time" that he enjoyed with his family.

VACATION NIGHT

Once you've eaten that dinner (again, we recommend consuming this between 6 PM and 7 PM), it's time to treat yourself. What?! Yes, that's right, treat yourself. Many people don't fast because they think it's hard and unpleasant. So they imagine that anyone who does must be having some kind of ascetic self-denial experience during which they walk around sulkily with a frown and indulge in their misery of not eating. This is simply not true.

One of the main reasons that you're going to succeed in your initial fast is because you're going to create and savor an enjoyable experience. A way to set this up is to transition out of the stresses of your day and into a relaxing evening. When I've had an intense day in the ER, I know I'm going to need to run or workout to blow off some steam so that I come into my pre-fast dinner and Vacation Night with the right mindset and commitment to relaxation.

To make sure I do this, I often text or call my wife, Regina, as I'm leaving the hospital and ask her to put my gym clothes and shoes outside the garage door. That way I have no excuse to skip my run. Sometimes she'll encourage me to load up my surfboard and follow the advice of Randy Rarick, who says that a good session involves "going out for an hour or at least catching three waves."[31] Randy makes sure he does this every day and finds it particularly helpful when he's in the middle of pro surfing's frenetic Triple Crown season. We encourage you to create a similar buffer between your work or school day and the first two stages of the fast. You need time to mentally and physically unpack the day and transition from a productive, task-oriented frame of mind to a more laidback one.

TIME TO TALK

My inspiration for the title of this chapter comes from the short getaways that Regina and I sometimes take by ourselves. While we enjoy spending family time with our sons, we also savor those few hours when it's just the two of us. Usually her folks come to our house to look after our kids, and we head out for a brief getaway. We'll put music on in the car and just enjoy the drive and being in each other's company. Sometimes we'll go for a walk along the beach or watch a movie. But some of our best Vacation Nights have been when we just talk.

For those few precious hours, I'm no longer an ER doctor and Regina isn't a physical therapist. We're no longer just parents. We're not the founders of VitalityPro. No. We're just good ol' Frank and Regina. Though we obviously have some dialogue every day during the week, these are often the kind of truncated conversations that all couples have in passing on their way to work, to kids' activities, or to social engagements. But it's on these Vacation Nights that we get to spend two, three, or more hours just talking—unpacking frustrations from the week that was, celebrating triumphs, recounting funny things our boys did or said. We don't bring tablets or laptops that would invariably distract us, and we resolve not to look at emails or texts or our phones. We only answer a call if it's from whoever's watching the kids. This is a way of protecting our time together.

One of my favorite books is *Boundaries*. In it, Dr. Henry Cloud and Dr. John Townsend give practical ways for you to get better at setting limits for yourself and others and tips for asking them to do the same for you. This was where I was introduced to the concept of safeguarding time. Sometimes that can be with my work. When I'm at the trauma center, a life literally depends on my focus on who and what is in front of me. So I can't be messing around with my phone as it would divert me from the very pressing task at hand. Or it could be the hours I spend taking our boys out into the waves at the beach. With the kids, Regina set me the boundary of putting my phone in the glove box when I'm coaching their soccer team. And as I had to be a proactive participant in running these sessions rather than just passively watching someone else do it, the coaching role was itself a boundary.

I extend the *Boundaries* philosophy to these brief escapes with Regina. Sometimes we see another couple at a table with glasses of wine and food in front of them and they're not even paying attention to each other. Why? Because they're engrossed in messing with their phones! Maybe you can take an honest look at yourself and see that you're one of those people. If you are, I implore you to read *Boundaries* and to start putting its lessons into practice.

You don't even have to wait that long to be more intentional, focused, and devoted to your relationships. We believe that by applying the same mindset Regina and I have on our Vacation Nights to the evening stage of your fast, you're going to improve the quality and extend the quantity of your time spent engaging with family and friends. Rather than flitting between tech distractions, work to dos, and all the other things that can so easily divert our attention, we want you to try and be fully and totally present with people for a change. This might be uncomfortable at first because you've conditioned yourself to become so used to trying to do "this, that, and everything" at once that it has become the norm. That's OK. I promise that if you just stick with it and keep devoting two, three, or four hours for one Vacation Night per week as part of your fast, you'll start to rewire your brain and reset your habits. At some point, it will just become part of how you live your life.

For award-winning producer and musician Peter Furler, setting aside a couple of hours each week isn't enough. "I have to take a day a week to dedicate to my family," Peter said. "It's a matter of self-preservation. It's tempting to do a little work or update my social media feeds, but when I resist these temptations I find I'm more rested and productive the next day. It's also a way for me to slow myself down. It's the same when I ride my motorcycle. Rather than thinking about the quickest way to get somewhere, I actually choose twisty, less traveled roads because they force me to slow down and appreciate the journey."[32]

Similarly, if those close to you have gotten used to you never being fully present, it's going to take them some time to adjust to this new, focused, engaged you. Months, years, or even decades of behavior patterns set the tone for not just how individuals act in isolation but how they interact with others. So their initial suspicion that you haven't really changed might take some time to undo. But they'll soon come around and appreciate the fact that you're now determined to make them your sole priority for those few hours. And we bet that they're going to want more.

On the flip side, once you start having these rich experiences and show your loved ones that you do actually care about them, you're going to want more too. You'll wonder why you let external distractions draw you away from being present, and you'll start reordering your life to create more space for this new-found, truly *quality* time. This is just one of the ways that *The 17 Hour Fast* can start to have positive ripple effects on the rest of your home, work, and social life even once you're done fasting.

When we talked about this with our friend Mac Powell, lead singer of the band Third Day, he said, "For me, fasting isn't just about food but giving up other things for a little while too. I often fail to realize how addicted I am to my phone and the internet. I can also get selfish with my time and just want to sit down and read a magazine quietly. But when I make the effort to put down that magazine, turn my phone off, and go play outside with my kids I always get far more out of it."[33]

If you're single and don't have a spouse or kids, you might be thinking all this has little or no relevance for you. Not so. Everyone has somebody in their life, whether it's parents, siblings, extended family, friends, or colleagues. Just because Vacation Nights typically involve our immediate family doesn't mean that it has to be the same for you. Maybe the relationship component of your night is getting together with some buddies to watch a ball game, going out with some coworkers, or driving across town to see a relative. Though we recommend putting aside technology for most of your evening, it's OK to use it to enhance, develop, or even fix a relationship. If you can avoid letting it take you down a post-conversation internet rabbit hole for the rest of the night, you could send a long, thoughtful email to a family member, rather than the usual two- or three-liners you usually dash off as you're clearing out your inbox. If you recently read on Facebook that a friend's wife is struggling with sickness or that your uncle lost his job, reach out to them and offer a listening ear. Or perhaps set aside time to call your grandma.

These are all appropriate, constructive, and intentional uses of technology that will not only improve relationships for you, but also for that other person. Maybe this initial contact is just the beginning of overcoming a feud, deepening a connection, or investing in a friendship that you've been neglecting recently. Too often we just think of investments as how much is in our retirement or kids' college savings account or get fixated on the values of our stocks and bonds. These are an important component of our financial lives, but they're not life itself.

Phil's a big fan of the BBC show *Sherlock*. One of the best bits of this show is when Sherlock tells his best friend John Watson, "Alone is what I have. Alone protects me." Watson, incensed, replies, "No, friends protect people." This is very true. When things go wrong in our lives, we need our friends and family members to protect us, offer comfort and advice, and get us through tough times. But we can't take them or this protection for granted. Just as you need to make regular contributions to your 401K and other fiscal accounts, so too do you need to make regular deposits in the lives of those around you. If you commit to investing in them, they'll invest in you too.

The trouble is that we get so caught up in our careers or school work, so focused on maintaining hundreds of followers and cyber friends on social media, and so lost in the fog of our crammed calendars that we lose sight of the people who are important. And they're not going to know that they matter to you unless you spend time—dialed in and devoted time—with them as often as you're able. The Vacation Night is your chance to restart your relationship investment strategy, which is far more important in the long run than your financial portfolio.

A VACATION NIGHT VICTORY

Our friend and minister, Jack Reece, encourages me as a father and husband by repeatedly saying, "There is no quality time without quantity of time." For Jack, fishing is the perfect venue for him to purposely create protected "quantity of time" for his special family members and friends. He encourages other parents to fish with their families as they have a captive audience while on the boat (and maybe because he loves fishing too).

Regina and I use some Vacation Nights as family time without any outlined activities. Sometimes impromptu nights are needed. Anyway, it was on one of those spontaneous evenings that I was tempted to be a hypocrite and sneak upstairs to outline this book's next chapter for Phil. Fortunately, our fun discussion at the table after dinner made me decide to honor that "quantity of time" that Jack's often reminding me about.

THE 17 HOUR FAST

Over the next hour, our boys' funny discussion transitioned into more thoughtful questions regarding our beliefs. Later, both of our boys accepted and made a lifelong commitment to our faith. It was one of the most joyous times for Regina and me.

Everyone has a faith or value system that is personal and important. As parents, we have such a short time to teach our children all of these guiding principles of life. In respect to your faith or belief system, my prayer is that each of us will prioritize creating protected family time and thus will experience such joyous occasions.

THE MEANING OF GAME NIGHT

If Regina and I aren't on one of our rare but precious overnight hotel stays or out with friends, we're usually doing things with our kids. If you have children too, you can turn this evening into a family-focused one. I try to throw a ball with my kids before the sun sets. After my final pre-fast meal, we then get the games out and play checkers for a couple of hours. Then Regina reads bedtime stories to all of us. Phil's family likes to play Scrabble, Uno, and Monopoly after a trip to the soccer field and the library. The activities you choose don't really matter, just as long as you're doing them together.

All too often we pay lip service to the fact that our kids are the most significant things in our lives as parents, but do we prove this in how we order our schedules? If your child is all excited to tell you about a top grade they got on a test, a new friend they made, or the game they won on the playground and you just tell them "uh-huh" as you stare at a screen, the light in their eyes grows dim. They assume that what they were so eager to tell you doesn't matter. If this is repeated often enough, perhaps they start to wonder if they matter.

We seem to have an epidemic-level struggle with attention deficit disorders in this country, and I'm far from the perfect parent. But when Regina and I take our kids to the beach or sit down to play a game with them, we don't just put our phones on silent or vibrate mode but actually turn them off. We're not going back and forth to our laptops every few minutes to check our email. And we recognize that while we sometimes post pictures of our boys, we're more focused on doing life with them than recording our experiences in photos and videos. This is another example of creating boundaries in our lives and giving them the same status as police "Do Not Cross" tape. If you let one text, email, social update, or phone call in, others will follow. This Vacation Night is your opportunity to pay more and better attention to your kids and to consciously block out all other diversions, until this becomes an unconscious rhythm and pattern in your life.

This topic brings me to a bigger point. It's very easy to identify several aspects of our lives and call them our top priorities. But the proof is in the calendar pudding. That doesn't sound very appetizing, does it? But joking aside, a quick test to see if we're living out our real priorities is to look at our calendars and see how we're allocating our time. Then think about the impact these scheduling choices have on those around us. As my father frequently told me, "When you say yes to something, that means you say no to something else." When we're continually saying yes to yet more work time and no to our spouse and kids, that's a problem. If we're devoting hours a day to staring at a screen and neglecting our friends because of it, we might need to rethink our time management.

I remember reading about Peyton Manning frequently taking his linemen out to dinner. He recognized that these were the guys who would determine the fate of his season, his career, and his health by either protecting his blind side when he was stepping back to throw or leaving him exposed to onrushing opponents. We probably aren't going to step out into the first down of a Super Bowl anytime soon, but like Peyton, we need people to look after us. The ones who should be defending our blind side and blocking the onrushing problems and difficulties that we all face in life should be our family and friends. Just like that legendary quarterback, we need to spend quality time with them so they know that they matter to us and will in turn show up when we need them to.

We also find that it's helpful during the evening to practice a little gratitude. In a couple of chapters' time, we'll discuss how this can set you up nicely for the Spa Morning phase of your fast, but it's also good to bookend the evening with it. If you have a family, maybe you each say a couple of things that you were thankful for that day. Should you be a person of faith, this can lead seamlessly into prayer, meditation, and the study of sacred texts. Or simply take a few minutes to be thankful.

GET COMFORTABLE WITH PAMPERING

One of the reasons I call this a "Vacation Night" is because when you are on vacation, you have the opportunity to actively cut yourself off from the usual distractions and influences of the outside world. You become totally engaged in the massage, sauna, face mask, or whatever other treatments you choose at the hotel spa or in the activities your destination has to offer. Even if you don't actually go on a mini-vacation for this first phase of your fast, you should try to create similar conditions. If you have a good massage therapist, go get a treatment from them. And if you're married, nothing gets you brownie points quite like giving the gift of a couples massage. It's also worth noting that a massage feels completely different when you're fasting because when you're "flex fueling" on ketones, your neurons are firing in a different way than when you're mostly relying on glucose.

You can also have the spa or movie theater come to you, even if this doesn't mean an in-home massage or manicure. If you're into movies, we know you have to skip the popcorn and snacks during your fast, but you could still get a rental or fire up Netflix and watch a film together. Or if you decide you want to go completely tech-free during this stage of the fast, you could dim the lights or get out that box of candles you haven't used in years to create a softer, more relaxing ambience (this is a contrast to harsh, white LED bulbs than can disrupt melatonin production). Into music? Then put on some tunes. Many people say they love music, but when was the last time you let an entire album play and listened intently to the lyrics or melody?

If you're not just a consumer of music but also a creator, then use this time to practice some riffs on your guitar, put all those years of piano lessons your parents made you do into practice, or dare we say, irritate your neighbors by blasting the dust off your drum kit. We get so wrapped up in the work element of the pursuit of happiness that we often lose sight of the actual "happy" part. In which case, you can utilize this Vacation Night to inject some fun back into your life.

We hope that you reach a ripe old age but nothing is for certain. In the emergency room, I see all too many young people whose time on this earth is cut tragically short by accidents and illness, and that has instilled a certain carpe diem (seize the day) spirit in me. We're not suggesting giving into reckless hedonism but rather saying that you shouldn't slave away every day so you can do things in a retirement that you don't know you'll see. Life is for living, and we hope you use this one night a week to start doing just that.

THE ACCOUNTABILITY ADVANTAGE

We've found that people who do their fasting with someone else typically have a higher success rate than those who go it alone. Research reveals that people who are trying to quit smoking or drinking alcohol are up to 400 percent more likely to do so if they have an accountability partner, and studies show that people stick to an exercise routine better if they have a buddy doing it with them. So if you can talk your better half into joining you in the fast and the surrounding experience, we encourage you to do that.

What's in it for them, other than giving you moral support? Well for starters, you can pamper them one night a week, which can become like another date (if you're as busy as my wife and me, I bet your relationship will benefit). Pitch it this way rather than focusing on the absence of food and you're more likely to bring them along for the ride. You could also get a friend or a whole group together to fast on the same night. Even if they can't be with you, you can still keep each other accountable and share hints, tips, and encouragement before and after your fast. I've had administrators, doctors, and nurses at my hospital, friends in the business world, and some of my pals who are first responders do the fast on the same night/morning as me, and I have found that we've benefited greatly from sharing our personal experiences.

REVERSING FOOD BRAINWASHING

Remember what we said in the introduction about using *The 17 Hour Fast* not merely as a method for improving your biology but also for rewiring your habits and motivations? Every day we're bombarded by messages telling us to eat more and make worse nutritional choices. The Rudd Center for Food Policy and Obesity found that the fast food industry spends $4.6 billion each year on advertising, while in the first two months of 2016 alone, snack food companies poured $100 million into TV advertising, not to mention the billions they spend annually on online ads.[34]

This adds up to us being systematically brainwashed into buying unhealthy food that's making us sicker than ever before. Advertising— whether delivered via traditional media like print and TV or online—is part of what's called the "attention economy," which is basically the monetization of capturing and holding our focus and converting this into purchasing. And then from there, one-time shoppers are turned into loyal repeat customers who habitually stop by the drive-through or the supermarket snack aisle on their way home from work every night.

Snack companies and fast food restaurants are continually upping their attention economy game and are driving the addiction component of it. Next time you watch a movie or sports game on TV, we encourage you to keep a tally. For every food-related ad you see, add a mark, and then at the end of the program, total them up. You'll be amazed by how many "eat" or "drink" messages you just got bombarded with.

Most of our major league sports now have TV timeouts so the networks can cram in more ads than ever before. And after the Super Bowl, much of the water cooler chatter in offices isn't about the game itself but rather the funny, creative, or just downright seductive commercials. And while Super Bowl ads get all the press, it would be foolish to think that those shown during the regular season aren't making an impact, even if this is mostly subconscious. You might have heard the old adage, "It takes seven impressions to make an impression." Well in sports games, advertisers are living that out. A survey conducted by Nielson and UBC found that the number of 30-second commercials in an average NFL telecast was 69.8, and this didn't even take into account shorter ad spots.[35] During the playoffs, this jumps to 112 ads per game, with 8 percent of these being beer commercials and 12 percent for junk food. That's 22 ads per game telling you to eat and drink more.

As it has taken years for our brains to become biased toward certain junk and fast food brands, it's going to require continued effort to free ourselves from this mind control. While you can't expect a complete change in mindset or habits overnight, you can use this Vacation Night to get started on the right road by avoiding TV, online, and print ads for junk food. If you can commit to doing *The 17 Hour Fast* once a week for a year, you're going to have 52 opportunities to rewire your brain and start creating replacement reward systems that aren't focused on food. That process starts tonight.

TUNING BAD NEWS OUT

In addition to avoiding food-related ads and sleep-disrupting blue light and creating a deeper engagement with family and friends, setting gadgets aside enables us to sidestep the pressures of work and the negativity of news media. You want this fasting journey to be a pleasant and positive one, so try to insulate yourself from negativity, cynicism, and external pressure from your boss, colleagues, or clients. If you watch a movie, try and make sure it's one that's funny or uplifting, rather than a film with a lot of violence or a tragic ending.

Avoid watching the news because the majority of it is negative and gets us all worked up. Shootings, wars, and natural disasters promote the kind of panic and anxiety we're trying so hard to avoid during this Vacation Night. If your stocks have taken a tumble, clicking over to a financial channel is going to get you all bent out of shape too. And don't get us started on divisive political commentators. We often overlook the powerful connection between the media we consume, our emotions, and the physiological response in our bodies and brains. This fast is a chance to acknowledge this and direct your mood positively.

RETHINKING HYDRATION, CAFFEINE, AND SLEEP AIDS

In addition to addressing our psychology, we need to think about our biology. We spend a lot of time, money, and effort revving ourselves up from the moment we get out of bed. For a lot of people, their first act is to turn on their coffee maker (I'm guilty of this), and the Starbucks drive-through is a daily detour on the way to work. Add in a couple of runs to the coffee shop later in the day and it's clear what the addiction of choice is in this country, to the tune of 3.1 cups per person per day and $40 billion a year. Phil admits to being guiltier than most on this front, though in his defense, he also says his home espresso machine played a big part in writing this book!

For some people, such natural caffeine isn't enough, so they turn to so-called energy drinks for an even bigger buzz. Now there's nothing inherently wrong with coffee, and goodness knows we like a cup of Joe as much as anyone. And in fact, there are many benefits, from improved concentration to enhanced fat metabolism to protecting the brain against the ravages of cognitive decline. But if we go overboard, the costs can soon start to cancel out some of these benefits. If we're always high on caffeine, we can exacerbate certain issues like high blood pressure. During our fast, we're trying to do the opposite of what we do when we stumble into the kitchen first thing in the morning and put a pot of coffee on.

The goal here is to slow down, cycle down, and calm down. That's why we recommend drinking water regularly and either avoiding caffeine altogether or, if you're hooked on it, tapering your consumption to half and drinking it earlier in the day. One of the reasons is that the half-life of caffeine (amount of time required to reduce the amount in your bloodstream by 50 percent) is around six hours for most people. It then takes an additional six hours for the caffeine to be halved again. During the fast, we want you to get the best quality sleep possible and if you're slugging a mug of coffee at 9 PM, you're still going to have half the caffeine in your system at 3 AM and will still have quarter of it at 9 AM. If you're a slower metabolizer of caffeine, the half-life might be an hour or two longer, increasing its sleep-disrupting effects.

Another substance we need to talk about is alcohol, which many people use as a natural sleep aid. It might make you drowsy and help you fall asleep but tends to negatively impact your second and third sleep phases. One issue with combining alcohol and fasting is that because alcohol is a depressant, your body may produce "excitatory" hormones to balance out that effect. As your body metabolizes the alcohol while excitatory hormones persist, this leads to an imbalance which disrupts your sleep. Again, I'm not going to act like a finger-wagging Puritan and say, "Thou shalt not consume any alcohol or caffeine." Instead of going cold turkey, if you enjoy an evening drink, I encourage you to taper the amount that you consume. And then make sure you savor that one glass, bottle, or can as you enjoy the company of a friend or family member, if you didn't already have it during your pre-fast dinner.

Sleep aids can also pose some challenges. An estimated 164 million Americans struggle to fall or stay asleep at least once a week and many have chronic issues with insomnia and other sleep disorders. Phil and I both have friends and family members who've dealt with such issues for years, and we feel bad for them. To try and overcome these issues, Americans are spending $41 billion a year on sleep aids, and this is projected to rise to $50 billion by 2020.[36] The fact that we're continuing to spend more and more on sleeping pills shows that we're not winning the war on sleep deprivation.

We'd never want to minimize or discount the significance of anyone's sleep issues or the fact that right now, they need the medicine that they're taking. But by creating a relaxing vibe during your Vacation Night and improving your sleep hygiene routine, you can help improve sleep duration and quality and enhance the positive effects of whatever sleep aid you might be taking. Even though it may take a few weeks or months, you will also likely experience less interruptions and disturbances. If you do start to get better rest and think you might like to change the dosage of a prescription, please talk to your doctor about this.

And now a word about natural sleep aids like melatonin. These can prove helpful as a temporary remedy but they are not a cure. If you are using something natural in an unnatural way, then it becomes unnatural. You need to start trying to change behavior to address the root of your sleep challenges, rather than just masking the symptoms or making them manageable.

That said, if you suddenly stop taking a natural or prescribed sleep aid altogether, you're probably going to toss and turn all night and wake up grumpy and frustrated. Instead, it's better to start slowly tapering your dose if your doctor or sleep therapist says it's OK. If you simply stop taking medication, you're creating a large difference between what you're used to and what you're now doing that's going to shock your system and do more harm than good. So make any change gradual.

RECONNECTING TO THE ELEMENTS

At the same time as you disconnect from technology during the Vacation Night, we want you to reconnect to something else: the natural elements. We've found that watching the sun set and then stargazing when it gets dark is one of the most effective ways to recalibrate the body with celestial and diurnal patterns. From a brain perspective, seeing darkness fall prompts you to make more sleep-inducing melatonin and reduce production of stimulating chemicals that keep you awake. Then there are the effects of looking up at the moon and stars. I started doing this more than a decade ago during my post-graduate research at Pepperdine University. It helped me understand the magnitude and complexity of creation and how small my problems were. After just a few minutes of staring up at the night sky, I'd invariably slip into sleep. The effect is just as profound today.

I also find it very relaxing to get into a body of water during the Vacation Night. For me, just wading out a little way into the Gulf of Mexico is one of the ultimate relaxation techniques. It's even more beneficial when I get out past the breakers and into calm waters. Then I just float on my back, letting go of all my tension and allowing the current to carry me. If you don't have access to the ocean, you could try a dip in your local lake or river if it's warm outside. No natural body of water nearby? Then maybe do a slow-speed swimming session or take a relaxing soak in a hot tub or bath. If you're going to start off in warm or hot water, get out before you start to feel a prickly sensation on your skin. Staying in any longer means that you've overshot the mark a little with the heat and have triggered a histamine response. We also recommend that you finish with some lukewarm or cool water. Opinions vary on the best duration for this, but in our research, we've found that a minute or a little less is all it takes to cool you down and trigger the positive effects of thermal therapy. Experiment a bit and find the protocol that is best for you.

You might also find that you like the sound of running water. Try getting a small fountain and putting it on your patio or in your backyard. If you place it outside your bedroom and leave the window cracked at night, you'll get the benefits of that soothing sound as you settle down for sleep.

Another natural element that can help us reconnect to nature and wind down during the Vacation Night is weather. Watching the snow fall or listening to the wind rustle the leaves of the trees in your neighborhood can be very meditative, if you allow yourself to focus on it for a few minutes. Feeling a snowflake land on your tongue or raindrops hit your head are two other simple ways to engage with the weather.

Getting out in and observing the weather improves our awareness of seasonal rhythms as well. We just covered how watching the sun set and staring at the stars and moon can help re-attune our senses to the circadian cycles of day and night. In our hustle and bustle, we also tend to overlook the changing of the seasons. Just like the opposition of day and night, the seasons were designed to provide a natural balance—hot and cold, sunshine and showers, longer and shorter days, and all the other contrasts that we see as spring, summer, fall, and winter blend into one another.

We sadly pay little attention to such transitions. Try to make a point of noticing the conditions of whatever season you find yourself in and then make a conscious effort to see slower changes as the weeks and months move ever onward. We think you'll find this contemplation to be deeply restorative.

BREAKING THE STRESS CYCLE

There are equally effective mechanisms in the brain that stimulate us (sympathetic nervous system) and calm us down (parasympathetic nervous system). The sympathetic nervous system helps us survive stress in our lives just as it allowed our ancestors to stay alive as hunter gatherers while on the lookout for lions, wolves, bears, and other predators. The sympathetic nervous system doesn't differentiate various types of stress, whether physiological or psychological.

But as a rule, we may be far worse than our ancient ancestors at balancing this out with the parasympathetic nervous response, which is designed to help us wind down, fully digest our food, and repair our bodies and minds from the stressors of each day. By the time we get to the evening, we're meant to be leaning more toward the parasympathetic end of things so we can process our dinner, enjoy social settings, and start preparing for restorative sleep.

Yet it's all too easy to shift quickly into high gear and much more difficult to move that shifter back down to neutral and then park. We've talked a little about how technology is partly responsible for keeping our minds stimulated around the clock, and we will be discussing further the role caffeine plays in our continually elevated state. When I decide to do *The 17 Hour Fast,* I make a conscious decision that every activity I engage in is going to chill me out, not rev me up.

One of the things we find helpful is to do some relaxed breathing work. At VitalityPro, we do what we call a "good night," which is the opposite of the "good morning" you might be familiar with if you've ever practiced yoga. It's basically a straight-leg toe touch, whereby you slowly breathe in as you stand straight up with arms stretched upward and then slowly breathe out on the way down. Each cycle is slower than the last one. You're welcome to try 10 or 20 of these during your Vacation Night and see how you feel afterward.

You can also do some controlled breathing, in which you take a slow nasal inhale and then exhale even slower through your nose. You'd be amazed by how beneficial this can be in turning off your stress mechanism. It's also effective to combine this with some mobility exercises, such as those featured in Dr. Kelly Starrett's book *Becoming a Supple Leopard*. Like Kelly, my wife, Regina, is a physical therapist who knows better than most how impactful doing some soft tissue work in the evening can be.

SETTING UP FOR SPA MORNING SUCCESS

Before you go to bed, spend a few more moments being proactive about your forthcoming Spa Morning. Set your alarm for 15 to 30 minutes earlier than usual so you won't need to rush in the morning. Sure, you'll lose a little sleep, but you can easily gain this back by turning in a bit before you normally would. Getting up early will help you to avoid dashing around as you might most mornings and will enable you to ease into the final two phases of the fast. You might also want to set out your workout clothes if you plan to be active and work attire if you'll have to go into the office in the morning. If you're going on a family outing, retrieve your kids' clothes from their closet, prepare lunch, and pack your cooler. Do as many things as you can to make the next morning easier, and do so at a slow and calm pace.

We then suggest you spend a little time reading, listening to soft, quiet music, or doing any other non-technology activity that you find relaxing. Then repeat the breathing exercises from earlier on and get into bed. Make sure your room is dark, that you've removed all electronic devices, and that the thermostat is set two degrees lower than normal or to a maximum of 68. If you don't have air conditioning and the house has heated up during a hot summer day, open some windows to make sure your body is at the optimal temperature for sleep. Live in a noisy location? Then use earplugs or a white noise machine to drown out distractions that might prevent you from falling asleep or wake you up in the middle of the night.

KETOTIC SLEEP

CHAPTER 7

This should be the easiest part of your fast, as you don't have to do anything except sleep. But there's more to the story. In this chapter, we'll be discussing the importance of proper sleep and the additive effect that a more balanced diet and fasting can have on your slumber.

The body needs to fuel the reparative functions that take place when we're sleeping. While eating the more ketotic pre-fast meals and fasting will help you switch from glucose-only fuel to a glucose/ketone blend, you'll never truly transition to 100 percent ketosis. Multiple studies and the work of experts like University of South Florida Molecular Pharmacology and Physiology professor Dominic D'Agostino show that having more ketones improves the quality of stage 3 sleep. This is when 80 to 90 percent of all growth and repair occurs.[37] In this chapter, we will share many tips that will improve the quality of your sleep, leading to better recovery of mind, body, and soul.

In our hectic culture, we've come to view rest and recovery almost as an inconvenience. We idolize hard-working leaders and business people who get by on very little rest, yet we conveniently forget that some of these over-achievers suffer from shortened lifespans or limited quality of life. Similarly, some people attempt to replicate the workouts of elite athletes with little or no regard for their precisely matched nutrition/recovery/sleep programs. A lot of research data suggests that many athletes are routinely overtraining, which contributes to poor performance, injury, or illness.

At the simplest level, overtraining means someone is exposing themselves to a greater training stimulus than they're recovering from. So the cure is either less training or better recovery, and the easiest win is with the latter. Whether your area is business, athletics, or a creative pursuit, gaining a sleep/recovery advantage is of utmost importance. Phil has had times in his writing career when he's been staring down a deadline and has stayed up until 2 AM or later 12 out of 14 nights. And during my medical residency, I pushed myself to the brink several times. We've learned that this is not sustainable and that the short-term gain is not worth the long-term loss. It's the tortoise-and-hare philosophy made manifest.

Your need for nightly restoration and repair is no less important than that of an elite athlete. Whether it's committing things we've learned during the day to long-term memory, buffering poor lifestyle choices, or repairing the muscle teardown that follows physical activity, sleep is a daily opportunity to start tomorrow better than we ended today. Sleep is the ultimate "reset" button.

SLEEP DEFICIT PROBLEMS

Opinions vary about how much sleep we should be getting, but it turns out that the good old eight hours we've been told about for years is pretty close to the mark (our research shows 7.7 hours, but let's not split hairs). A bit more is fine, and some people need more recovery because of their higher output. LeBron James and Roger Federer reportedly get nine or ten hours a night. But while some of us can thrive on more than eight hours, most of us can't be our best if we get much less. Once we dip below a seven-hour average, we start to see some issues developing. Due to a reduction in metabolic activity, people who get chronically poor sleep have a higher incidence of obesity. This in turn raises the risk of sleep apnea, which further compromises sleep.

In addition to this vicious cycle, getting less than seven hours every night is also strongly linked with an increased likelihood of cardiovascular disease and metabolic syndromes. It also appears to aggravate a lot of digestive issues. The rates of type 2 diabetes are higher among poor sleepers, and inadequate sleep correlates with a higher incidence of hypertension and elevated LDL and total cholesterol. And as we explored earlier, if you have diabetes, high blood pressure, and high cholesterol, you're at far greater risk of suffering from the three main types of atherosclerotic issues: heart disease, stroke, and peripheral vascular disease. Studies that have compared day- and night-shift workers who get the same amount of sleep have uncovered that the night workers have a higher risk of developing cardiovascular disease, type 2 diabetes, and many other conditions than those who work during the day.

An international research team led by Dr. Jean-Claude Marquié from the University of Toulouse discovered that ten years of rotating shift work has the equivalent effect on the brain of six-and-a-half years of cognitive decline.[38] The work of Marquié and other researchers also demonstrates that shift workers and people who are sleep deprived also score much lower on cognitive and memory tests. They recover more slowly from illness and injury and have diminished muscle growth and repair as well.

Sleep deprivation can also disrupt the balance of sex hormones, such as testosterone and estrogen. This can contribute to conditions like low testosterone or infertility in men and polycystic ovarian syndrome in women. Other hormones that see alterations include cortisol, epinephrine, norepinephrine, serotonin, GABA, and dopamine. As a result, sleep-challenged folks can be more emotionally labile, and sleep deprivation can be a contributing factor to some psychiatric conditions, including anxiety and depression-related disorders. Simply put, getting inadequate sleep once in a while isn't going to kill you. But if this becomes an issue night after night, it very well may. At the least, you'll have a diminished quality of life and a whole host of physical, cognitive, and emotional challenges that are perfectly avoidable if only you increased the quality, duration, and consistency of your sleep.

THE SLEEP STAGES

Even though this isn't a sleep book, having a basic understanding of sleep physiology gives us a better understanding and makes the tips and techniques in this chapter more useful. Here's a quick overview of the sleep stages.

In addition to the REM (rapid eye movement) stage, there are three stages of non-REM (NREM) sleep in each sleep cycle:

STAGE 1 NREM: You're just starting to drift off to sleep. This is when you might experience some myoclonic jerks, which is a fancy name for the muscle contractions that can half wake you up. It's easy to be awoken by noise or other sensory stimuli during this stage.

STAGE 2 NREM: In this second phase, you begin drifting into a deeper sleep and are less aware of sounds that may have awoken you during stage 1. Your heart rate and body temperature begin to drop.

STAGE 3 NREM: Now you're in a much deeper sleep stage, where most of your growth, repair, and replenishment occurs, both physically and cognitively. This is the stage that ketosis, or at least having a slightly higher percentage of ketones in your blood, can enhance. Breathing rate, blood pressure, and heart rate are all at their lowest point during this third stage. Much of our stage 3 sleep occurs earlier in the night during the first two sleep cycles.

REM STAGE: As the name suggests, your eyes move rapidly during this fourth and final stage. Your muscles are relaxed, and you're more likely to remember dreams. REM sleep typically accounts for 20 to 25 percent of all sleep, though the amount reduces with age. As we move closer to waking, we're in REM more than the other three stages. Breathing is more irregular in this stage, and blood pressure and heart rate are higher.

We've found that the first two full sleep cycles are crucial and that getting them completed as early in the night as possible has a lot of value. This is because we're meant to align our sleep habits with the natural rhythm of day transitioning into night. Being synchronized with the universe has its benefits.

Now this is not to say that being an early bird is inherently virtuous or that being a night owl is bad. We know from Michael Breus's book *The Power of When* that we all have slightly different chronobiology. But if you're at the late end of the scale and have any choice in the matter (i.e., you don't have to work late or deal with a crying newborn baby), you should try to go to bed a bit earlier and see if you feel more rested in the morning.

Anyway, back to the sleep stages. As we move through the night, the depth at which we go down into each stage diminishes. The time we spend in each one is also reduced, with the exception of REM sleep, which gets longer.

Children typically spend far more time in stage 3 NREM sleep than adults do, particularly when compared to elderly people. This is probably because their growing bodies and minds are driving the replenishment that occurs here. If we continue to challenge our bodies through physical exertion and our minds through new skill acquisition and development, we may begin to naturally spend more time in the reparative stage. This is not to say that we're going to stop or reverse aging. But going back to the idea we shared earlier about demand driving supply, we can partake in physical and mental activities that require greater restoration and growth. This has the potential to improve the quality of our sleep and, therefore, our vitality.

SYNCHRONIZING THE FAST AND SLEEP TO NATURE'S PATTERNS

Back in our "hunter and gatherer" days, our ancient ancestors would be out all day hunting, fishing, and foraging for berries and plants. Their life was work first and eat later if they were successful. This pattern of ancient life imprinted a biological design into hormonal and other physiological systems and set the diurnal release of hormones. It also established their complex positive and negative feedback interactions. In other words, our bodies developed and adapted their processes in conjunction with delayed and interrupted eating patterns.

Adipose (fat) tissue, which is viewed negatively in today's world, actually has many useful purposes—including insulation against cold and energy storage—when kept in proper balance. If we understand the biological processes governed by the endocrine system that use or convert adipose, we can use them to our advantage. That's why we have carefully synchronized (time shifted) 17 hours of fasting to match hormone patterns, including those that regulate cortisol, melatonin, and many others. Synchronizing the fast with these physiological systems enables you to get a better sleep that enhances hormone balance and release.

So what happens to these hormones when you're sleeping? First let's look at ghrelin. It's called the "hunger hormone" because, well, it makes you hungry. Ghrelin is made in the stomach and increases when the stomach is empty and less active. The good news is that ghrelin levels tend to decrease as you drift off to sleep.

Now let's shift our focus to leptin. This chemical is made by adipose tissue. Leptin goes up to the brain, where it helps suppress hunger via the arcuate nucleus within the hypothalamus. Remember, the hypothalamus is a region of the brain that acts like a big thermostat, regulating and balancing the many complex systems of the body. And just like the thermostat in your house, the hypothalamus takes in information from the body and then makes the necessary adjustments. If someone becomes obese, the abundance of adipose cells makes an abundance of leptin, which informs the hypothalamus to suppress appetite. Likewise, if someone is underweight, the lack of adipose results in a lack of leptin, increasing appetite and hopefully restoring a healthy body weight. Adequate sleep increases levels of leptin, which can help suppress the desire to eat and help you improve your BMI score.

LEPTIN RESISTANCE

Even as the hypothalamus and endocrine system are working to create balance through these positive and negative feedback loops, the combination of obesity and chronic continuous eating will override such systems. One example is "leptin resistance." The leptin thermostat in the arcuate nucleus is kept sensitive and accurate by appropriately spaced eating habits, which closely follow leptin's message to reduce food intake. This lower food intake results in less adipose tissue, leading to less leptin. It's these low levels of leptin that restore the thermostat's sensitivity to it. As we override this system with continual food intake, obesity, and chronically elevated levels of leptin, the arcuate nucleus loses its sensitivity. People who are overweight or obese have leptin resistance (insensitivity), the same way a diabetic has insulin resistance (insensitivity).

However, when we get enough high-quality sleep, we can start to make an impact on such hormonal perfect storms. We've already seen how slumber decreases hunger-promoting ghrelin. Well, on the flipside, it also increases hunger-suppressing leptin. If you're overweight, we believe that by achieving better sleep you'll help get your hormone levels back in check at night, which can only have a positive ripple effect in the daytime. Also, through the fast itself and more so the portion control and improved food choices you're making for your pre- and post-fast meals, you'll start to reset your hormone balance by changing what and how often you eat. Such healthy habits can carry over well beyond the fast and start to become your new normal.

RESTORING GROWTH AND SEX HORMONES

Appropriate sleep not only restores "hunger hormones" to a premium balance but also improves regulation of other hormones that dictate physical and cognitive repair and recovery. If we're getting at least seven hours of premium sleep, testosterone appropriately increases in both women and men (yes, women need naturally appropriate levels of testosterone too). This prompts soft tissue repair when we're injured and muscle hypertrophy (increase in size) and restoration after exercise. Growth hormone levels also leap during adequate sleep—again, providing that we're getting enough shut-eye, that those hours are relatively uninterrupted, and that we're not affecting our sleep cycles with caffeine or alcohol.

There are men who suffer from conditions such as hypogonadism, where the testes don't make enough testosterone. Such people should be taking supplemental testosterone to re-establish normal physiological levels. Ketotic sleep alone is unlikely to replace doctor-guided supplementation but should be viewed as a technique to use in conjunction with such therapy. Yet for most healthy males, testosterone supplementation is likely unnecessary and could prove harmful in the long run. If you don't struggle with a serious testosterone-related condition, see if ketotic sleep allows you to re-establish a healthy balance of male hormones and increases your vitality.

"OK, Dr. Merritt," you say, "but how does this relate to sleep?" Well, if we want to boost the levels of growth hormone and testosterone to improve workout gains, speed recovery, and promote repair, we should look at what we can do naturally. In the case of these hormones, we know that exercise boosts them. By tearing down our muscles, taxing cardiovascular, pulmonary, and other systems throughout the body, and introducing an appropriate demand stimulus, we're forcing ourselves to adapt at the cellular level. Our cells cannot stay at the same baseline of function and deal with the demand stimuli of running, surfing, lifting weights, or whatever else we've done to challenge their status quo. The issue is that many of us aren't getting enough sleep and whatever ZZZs we do grab aren't of a high enough quality. Once again, studies show the restoration of adequate sleep increases levels of testosterone and growth hormone.[39]

We just spent a few paragraphs talking about men, but this isn't a guys-only book. We hope it doesn't sound like pandering when we say that women are more complex than men in many good ways, and one of these is hormonally. That said, the balance between estrogen, progesterone, etc. is an extremely intricate one. We're not going to dive into a deep explanation of how better sleep as part of *The 17 Hour Fast* can help you overcome a specific hormone-related condition. But having spent time creating this system with several excellent endocrinologists, we can confidently say that ensuring proper duration and quality of sleep can only help aid in restoring hormonal balance. If you have more questions, we suggest that you do some further reading on this topic and talk to your OB/GYN. Then see what positive changes you notice once you've been doing *The 17 Hour Fast* weekly for a couple of months.

SLEEP HYGIENE

Creating better "sleep hygiene"—the habits, routines, and environment that either help or hamper sleep—is key. By establishing an atmosphere of calm and relaxation during your Vacation Night, you're already ahead in the race to get better sleep. You set your alarm a little earlier so you can ease into the Spa Morning without the usual mad rush out the door. Hopefully this encourages you to go to bed a bit earlier (and if it doesn't, then I advise turning in thirty minutes earlier next time). Other relaxation techniques and tactics outlined in the last chapter, such as breathing, mobility, playing games, and reading, all promote a restful slumber. Avoiding the blue light from screens, which suppresses melatonin and increases alertness, and making sure your bedroom is cool will also help optimize your sleep (remember, bears hibernate in the winter and the Merritts sleep in 64 to 68 degrees F temperatures), as will avoiding caffeine and exercising late in the evening. Hopefully, all this leads to a good night's sleep with increased time in stage 3 NREM sleep, increasing and balancing important hormones, leading to better repair and restoration.

DEALING WITH WAKEFULNESS

If you have trouble falling or staying asleep—whether it's occasional insomnia or a chronic issue you've been struggling with for years—we hope that the calming effects of the Vacation Night and ketosis itself will help you start to overcome these difficulties. But despite the sleep-enhancing promise of ketotic sleep, it's not always smooth sailing when you first start to fast. We've read some reports in fasting books about getting clammy or sweaty during extended fasts of 24 to 48 hours or longer. That's another reason our fast is only 17 hours long and why we synchronized the start of it with a delicious supper that transitions smoothly into sleep.

There might be some anecdotal evidence, but no impactful studies have found such a causative link between fasting and serious sleep disruption. That said, a few people find that when they're entering a state of ketosis for the first time or two, they may have a little insomnia or restlessness. As anyone who has battled with such issues can tell you, this is highly frustrating and creates anxiety that makes it hard to go back to sleep. But only if you let it. In case you wake up during the sleep stage of your fast, we suggest keeping a book beside your bed so you can read for a few minutes before trying to fall asleep again.

You could also get out of bed and go grab a glass of cold water. This is one way to cool yourself internally. We've talked a bit about the importance of not being too hot at night. If you've already got your thermostat set in the high to mid 60s and still wake up too hot, consider changing your sleepwear and altering your bedding so you have less layers and bulk around and on top of you. It can also make quite a big difference whether you're wearing socks or not and how thin and breathable they are.

We often underestimate our body's ability to control temperature, so even if you make some of these adjustments and feel a little chilly, you're going to warm yourself up enough. This is why Phil's dad never used a hot water bottle as the rest of the family did during cold winter nights in England—he always said he preferred "to warm up naturally," and that's exactly right. Not that a hot water bottle can't be comforting, but most people don't need artificial heat unless they have some kind of condition that affects thermoregulation. For everyone else, let your body do what it does in regulating your core temperature.

Another tip to get back to sleep if you wake up during the night is to try breathing in slowly from your diaphragm and exhaling even slower—say a five-second nasal inhale with a seven- to ten-second nasal exhale. When many people try this for just five minutes, they find it makes them relax and feel sleepy. Brian Mackenzie has also found a lot of benefits from a breathing protocol with the inhale-breath hold-exhale ratio of 1:3:2. This means that for every second you take on the inhale, you multiply it by three for the hold and by two for the exhale. Try starting off with a four-second inhale, twelve-second breath hold, and eight-second exhale, all through your nose. Too difficult? Then dial the numbers back a bit. Or if such calculations wake you up more, simply breathe in and out through your nose slowly without timing. This almost always works for us. The key with wakefulness during the night is to not freak out because you're conscious. Try to remain calm, do something relaxing, and be thankful for a few extra minutes of time to reflect, pray, or meditate.

In our metrics-obsessed culture, it's all too easy to reduce sleep to a single data point: number of hours. While this is certainly one way to quantify sleep, we're doing ourselves and our much-needed slumber a disservice if this is the only way that we assess it. As with any piece of information, we can't merely look at this sleep total in isolation, but need to put it into a meaningful and broad context.

We can start by being more honest and accurate in our self-appraisal. Many people who track their sleep do so inaccurately because of the human tendency to exaggerate. I could say I go to sleep at 10 PM every night, but if I'm just getting into bed then and it takes me 15, 30, or even 45 minutes to drift off, then claiming that I got eight hours because I slept until 6 AM is wrong. We also fail to take into account the quality of our sleep. Smart watches, phone apps, and fitness trackers purport to monitor this for us, but how they're calculating their sleep scores remains a mystery locked inside an algorithm. If you're trying to evaluate the quality of your sleep, I'd begin by asking yourself a simple question: "Did I feel well rested when I got up this morning?" If so, then good for you! But if not, then we've got some work to do.

We also caution you against putting too much emphasis in activity trackers and apps that "measure" the quality of your sleep as well as the quantity. Some of these claim to know how long you spend in each sleep phase as well. Again, this technology gives your sleep a single score, often out of 100. We know plenty of people who've tried tracking their sleep this way, and you know what? They sometimes feel lousy when they get a high sleep score for the previous night and great on other mornings when their sleep score is much lower. Just as discussed in the book *Unplugged*, it's all about how you use and find benefit from technology.

What we suggest is following some of the tips in this chapter, reading other books on sleep and chronotherapy, such as Dr. W. Chris Winter's *The Sleep Solution* and Kat Duff's *The Secret Life of Sleep,* and putting what you learn into practice. Just as with nutrition and exercise, one size does not fit all when it comes to sleep. Do some trial and error to see what works and what doesn't. Again, your first fast might not provide your best sleep ever, but if you keep tinkering with your sleep hygiene while fasting weekly, we think you're going to achieve premium level rest that makes you feel great in the morning.

SPA MORNING

CHAPTER 8

You've made it through the first two phases of *The 17 Hour Fast.* Well done! In fact, when you consider that you spent two, three, or four hours on your Vacation Night and another eight in ketotic sleep, you're actually 60 to 70 percent of the way to the finish line. Now let's move into the penultimate stage—the Spa Morning. In the coming pages, we're going to cover some ways to maintain the sense of calm you created last night, to devote more time to growing yourself and your relationships, and to set a positive physical, mental, and spiritual tone for the rest of the day. You'll also discover a few things that you might find unconventional, most notably the concept of caloric redistribution to help others in need. But we promise we're not going to go all hippie-dippy on you; these concepts, which are backed by psychology studies, will be beneficial if you give them a chance.

THE END OF RUSH HOUR

Think about your usual morning routine for a minute and write down three words that describe how you feel. We bet some variation of "rushed," "stressed," or "anxious" was in the mix somewhere. In the chaos of modern life, it's hard enough to get ourselves out the door and on the way to work, school, or whatever we'll be doing that day in a timely manner. Then we add in the needs of our spouses and, if you're in the same blessed life stage we are, a couple of kids who need us to pack their lunch, make their breakfast, brush their teeth, and umpteen other things before we all pile into our car and get going.

As a result, our morning routine is often anything but routine—rather a jumbled, frenetic, rush-fest that closely resembles a high-intensity gym workout or, depending on how unruly the kids are being, an obstacle race through Lego bricks and school clothes. Sometimes we don't even have time for that morning cup of coffee. If we don't skip breakfast entirely, it's a hastily poured bowl of cereal or a piece of toast on the way out the door. And where on earth did we put those infernal car keys?

If any of this sounds even vaguely familiar, that's fine. You're not alone. That was how we used to live too. Honestly, that type of stressed lifestyle tries to creep back in from time to time. Fortunately, developing and applying concepts of *The 17 Hour Fast* to our lives helps us avoid many of the pitfalls of the "rush hour" lifestyle now. As a mentor told me, "If you fail to plan, you plan to fail." Let's develop a plan to succeed. To begin, here are some techniques and concepts that we can use during and outside of *The 17 Hour Fast*.

EARLY BIRD

What we need to do is to back up and change how we start the day. We've found that people have a far better experience and much greater chance of finishing their fasting if they continue the relaxation of the previous evening into what we call a Spa Morning. Rewinding briefly to the Vacation Night, an important preemptive step is to set your alarm 15 to 30 minutes earlier than usual. Yes, you just read this a few pages ago, but it bears repeating. For those dealing with chronic sleep-related issues, this might not be doable right away, but is still a worthwhile goal to work toward. If you went to bed at whatever is a reasonable time for you, then you should feel fairly well rested and waking up an additional quarter or half an hour earlier will help you reap more benefits.

Getting up earlier will help alleviate the sense of feeling rushed, hurried, and overwhelmed that is often a defining characteristic of many mornings and a big reason that 53 percent of Americans report missing breakfast at

CHAPTER 8: SPA MORNING

least once a week and 31 million rarely eat it at all—though not in the same intentional, positive way as you are during this fast.[40] And in fact, many of those who do eat breakfast aren't doing so in a manner that does them any favors. Of the 10,000 people surveyed by Instantly, 45 percent said they get their breakfast from a fast food drive-through, while half of those who eat their first meal of the day at home do so "on the run" as they're dashing out the door.[41] Many more turn to sugary cereals for their "most important meal of the day."

We don't just want to think about what we're *not* eating during the fast but how we can improve our breakfast habits tomorrow and every day after that. Is what we're putting into our bodies hurting or helping? Are we taking time to chew each bite enough so our bodies can fully digest our food? And are we letting ourselves get pulled into the internet whirlpool from the moment we get up or thoughtfully making time to focus on our family as we eat together first thing in the morning? The very act of asking ourselves these questions can help us improve our routine.

One of the best examples of someone who starts each day early with intentionality is Randy Rarick. Here's how he described his typical morning when he's not traveling for work:

"I get up and make myself a cup of tea. Then I go outside and watch the ocean for 10 or 15 minutes to see what the conditions are like. Some people charge out there as part of what we call the 'dawn patrol,' but I know that they're very aggressively going after waves so they can be done and get to work or wherever. So many years ago I decided I was going to wait a couple of hours and be part of the 'second shift.' Once I've spent that time looking at the ocean, I'll go back inside and get the newspaper and read it for a while. Then I head down to the beach around 8 or 8:30 AM. After I've attached my leash, I don't rush out into the surf. Instead I'll swim out 30 or 40 yards, dragging my board behind me. It lets me get in tune with the conditions and ease into the waves. Once I've got an hour in and at least three good waves, I feel a sense of accomplishment. I have started my day communing with nature and have done something to keep me fit. Then I'm happy to go and shape a board, make some calls, and catch up on some emails."[42]

PACE YOURSELF

We believe it's also beneficial to continue what you started during the Vacation Night and steer clear of news and social media. You can undo hours of positivity with a few seconds of exposure to disasters, bad news, and cynicism, so try to reinforce that boundary during your Spa Morning. And if you start checking email, you're inevitably going to short-circuit the slowdown that we're aiming for in this portion of *The 17 Hour Fast* as you get pulled back into meeting invites, work to-dos, and social RSVPs. That's not where you want to go during this protected time.

For greater insight on changing the pace of life for the better, we again turned to Randy Rarick:

> "I decided a long time ago that I wasn't going to run unless I'm late for a plane. Whatever I'm trying to get to is still going to be there if I take my time. That means that even when I'm busy, I never have to hurry. One time I was invited to an event in Peru and they had a surfer from each decade compete in a prone paddling race. Fred Hemmings was the guy from the 60s, and they chose me for the 70s. I started out pretty well, but then the young guys began passing me. Some of them got to the buoy where we were supposed to turn before I even made it halfway. By the time I got to the finish line on the beach, the winner was already having his celebratory drink. I ended up in last place, but while some people might get upset with themselves, I was OK with that. It's been a good metaphor for my life. I'm pretty mellow, and I've realized that I don't have to win. I just want to enjoy participating and take my time."[43]

Let's try to apply what Randy is teaching here about pace of life to your self-reflection time. We need to think intentionally about what we are focusing on. And for at least the first 30 to 60 minutes of the day, we want that to be yourself. First thing in the morning, we often get so worked up that it's hard to be present at all. The concerns of the day—that late morning meeting with your boss, the big project that you need to hit hard that afternoon, and the kids' sports games that evening—quickly pull our thoughts to 101 external things. As a result, we start the day looking outward when really, we should carve out time to begin by turning our gaze inward.

That sounds a little New Age, doesn't it? Well maybe it is, but if you look at cultures and religions around the world, you'll see millions of people who begin each morning with some kind of mindfulness or prayer practice. Yet we've come to view slowing down and taking time to reflect on our lives and our place in the universe as an unnecessary luxury that prevents us getting to the next item on our endless task list. We're so consumed with looking outward at what's right in front of us—our screens, our jobs, the things we want to buy, and so on—that we neglect to look upward and inward. We need to rediscover the value of being totally present for a few minutes a day and just concentrate on being, rather than doing. The fast is the perfect chance to start cultivating such a daily practice.

THE BREATH OF LIFE, THE BREATH OF CALM

There are many ways to enhance your health, but none are more important than improving your ability to breathe. Likewise, there are many techniques used to reduce anxiety and create calm but none as simple and yet as effective as a nice deep breath. Brian Mackenzie has "Art of Breath," and we at VitalityPro have "Pulm-Max." Even though our modalities/techniques differ, we both agree that breathing is "the low-lying fruit" of health and performance.

There are many different breathing techniques you could pursue. But for first thing in the morning, we like the "Genesis breath" the

BRUSH AWAY BAD BREATH

One of the common side-effects people report when fasting is bad breath, or halitosis. There are many suggested theories as to the source of this. While opinions vary on the exact source of "fasting halitosis," the remedy is simple and obvious—brush your teeth, tongue, and mouth (avoid chewing gum).

best. This involves simply taking a long, fast nasal inhale and then breathing out slowly through your mouth. Repeat this breath several times, breathing deeper with each cycle. This should be done at a slow, calm pace without hyperventilation. This has the effect of creating a lot of negative intrathoracic pressure, which brings more air into the lungs. Less known is that this greater negative pressure also increases the venous blood flow into the thorax, which "pre-loads" blood volume to the heart. This in turn improves cardiac output. A friend asked once, "Is this a good thing?" Yes, it's a very good thing. This improves both your breathing and circulation, while making them more efficient. In addition, combining breath work and meditation has been shown to deliver a whole host of health-promoting benefits, including stress management, improved cognitive function, and blood pressure reduction.

WATER IS LIFE

The behavioral psychologists who helped us develop and refine *The 17 Hour Fast* know that if we're going to stop performing one destructive habit, we need to replace it with the reward of another. As you won't be triggering a food-based neurochemical rush during this Spa Morning, we suggest replacing it with one of the most fundamental needs we have as human beings: water. We've talked a little about the benefits of thermal therapy—exposing the outside of our bodies to hot and cold to reset our nervous system, balance specific hormones, and relax us. Think of drinking a glass of cold water as thermal therapy for your insides. Feel the cooling sensation—which you normally wouldn't notice in your morning rush—as the liquid runs down your esophagus and the splash as it hits your empty stomach.

We know some friends who like to add a squeeze of juice from an organic lemon to flavor their water. Yes, it's a couple of calories but perfectly permissible during the fast. Personally, I like to walk outside to my garden and pick a couple of fresh spearmint and peppermint leaves. When I get back to the house, I rub them between my fingers, take time to smell the fresh fragrance, and then drop them into a glass of cool water. Adding mint and/or citrus juice can help combat the bad breath some people experience during a fast.

We also advise making a little investment in a filtration system. This could be one of those under-sink setups on your kitchen faucet, a two-stage refrigerator filter, or just a Pur or Brita jug. Water is the most abundant element on this planet, and our bodies are 50 to 75 percent water. So it's important that we're not just staying hydrated but also are taking in high quality, contaminant-free water. Water expert Bobby Boucher from the comedy *The Waterboy* says we need more "high quality H2O," and he should know. Thus, getting a filter is one of the most important upgrades you can make to your home.

Another benefit of drinking water is that it can help you feel a little satiety, even though your stomach is actually empty. Now there's no need to freak out here even if you are getting a bit hungry. Remember that you ate a nutritious meal yesterday evening, and if you're like many people, you might often miss a meal or two each week anyway. Hormonally, one of the reasons for hunger pangs starting up in the morning is that cortisol, which was at its lowest ebb overnight, is now rising and, if you get up at 5 AM like I usually do, typically peaks around 9 AM. More cortisol equals more hunger. Growth hormone, which is an appetite suppressant, peaked overnight—especially during ketone-enhanced stage 3 sleep—but is now dipping again. And the hunger hormone ghrelin is starting to make a comeback. So yes, your hormones are conspiring against *The 17 Hour Fast* at this point! But drinking plenty of water can help and so can taking your mind off your stomach.

HARNESSING THE POWER OF SOUND

After you first get out of bed and drink that refreshing glass of water, I want you to start the morning off well by putting on some music that you find relaxing. For me, that's classical, even though I'll admit that I'm a big rock fan the rest of the day. So I tune into one of Pandora's playlists in that genre. Phil usually chooses some downtempo electronic music, like his go-to album by BT, *This Binary Universe.* Whatever your musical taste is, choose something that's going to put you in a contemplative state of mind, rather than tracks that are going to get you all pumped up.

In addition to putting you in the right mood, there's a lot of evidence to show that music enhances memory, concentration, learning, and a whole host of other cognitive functions. For example, the authors of a Stanford

University School of Medicine paper noted that the brains of participants who listened to a symphony were actually changing in real time; this enhanced their ability to anticipate events and sustain attention.[44] There are even websites that serve up music designed to make you more productive, like www.focusatwill.com and www.brain.fm, which also offers curated selections for relaxing. If you're going to be reading or writing, listening to music without words will help you focus because the language centers in your brain won't be confused by two disparate word flows.[45]

Music can also positively impact your wellbeing. In a meta review of over 400 studies, McGill University neuroscientist and author of the fascinating book *This Is Your Brain on Music,* Daniel J. Levitin found that patients with anxiety disorders who listened to music daily lowered their cortisol levels more than those who took anti-anxiety medication. This is not an indictment of such pharmaceuticals but rather an illustration of how powerful music can be. He also discovered a strong correlation between music and the antibody immunoglobin A, which plays an important role in the effectiveness of the immune system.[46] If you play an instrument, this may have even greater brain benefits. A study published in *The Journal of Neuroscience* found that kids who played an instrument for two years greatly improved their language skills.[47] So that's my excuse for tormenting my family while trying to master Pearl Jam riffs on the guitar during some Spa Mornings!

IN SEARCH OF SUNLIGHT

In the Vacation Night chapter, we suggested watching the sun set and star gazing to help regulate neurochemicals like serotonin and melatonin that govern the diurnal rhythms of wakefulness and sleep, respectively (serotonin during the day related to sunlight and melatonin at night related to darkness). On the other end of the scale is the morning. One of the best ways to wake yourself, particularly if you're tired, is to get outside in full sunlight and spend at least 20 minutes outdoors. If you can take a stroll along the beach, on a trail, or through a city park, you'll get the double benefit of adding exercise into the equation, while walking to a coffee shop to get a little espresso (Phil made me put this in—he has a problem) completes the trifecta of sunshine, physical activity, and caffeine.

When I was in my medical residency many years ago, I once worked 143 hours in a week. That's not a "look at how hard working I am" badge of courage, but rather an extreme example of how work can intrude on your life. Since then, I've done many overnight shifts in the ER. When trying to transition between normal nighttime sleep to working all hours of the night and back again, I've found that other than fasting, daytime sunlight exposure is the most effective reset button out there. Even if you don't have to pull "all-nighter" work shifts or, if you're a student, all-night study sessions, you'd still do well to get out in the bright light of day during your Spa Mornings and other days of the week. You'll not only feel more alert but will unintentionally help improve the quality and duration of your sleep as well.

HOW'S YOUR SELF-INVESTMENT PORTFOLIO PERFORMING?

Instead of doing more work so you can buy more stuff or pad your retirement account, invest in your wellbeing for a change. Eliminate distractions and allow yourself to be fully present. If you're a person of faith, this can include reading your holy text and praying. If not, maybe you can reread the writing of a favorite author or poet.

Or if you're someone who's into nature, do what we suggested in the In Search of Sunlight section and make your meditation a walking one in which you try extra hard to pay attention to the sights, sounds, and smells of whatever natural environment you can find. We know that not everyone gets to live in the mountains or by the ocean. But even if you're in a city, you can likely take a walk by a river, reservoir, or canal or locate some green space to explore. There are also meet-up groups like Walk2Connect and Mappy Hour in many cities, which encourage like-minded people to get together and enjoy being outdoors.

Perhaps you once journaled or kept a diary and abandoned the practice when being busy got the best of you. Now is a good time to rediscover this helpful habit. Other people compose positive affirmations, brainstorm to help solve a particular problem, or just write down whatever comes into their heads in the moment. None of these disciplines is necessarily better or worse than another. The key is finding something—reading, contemplating, journaling, painting, and so on—that encourages you to look inward and let the hustle and bustle of life fade into the background for once. Mac Powell revealed that when he gets back from a tour, he makes a concerted effort to ask himself some tough questions. "It's too easy to lose sight of your priorities, so periodically I need to think, 'Why am I doing this?' and 'What's my purpose?'" Mac said. "Fasting makes space for this kind of deep introspection that you don't get when you're caught up in everyday routines."[48]

In this Spa Morning phase, it's crucial to keep the calm, positive mood that you achieved the previous night going. Try to smile and laugh a lot as your attitude will largely dictate how you feel for the remainder of the fast. Should you wake up 30 minutes to an hour earlier than usual, our advice is to go with what your body's doing and get up. Make breakfast for your family—though not yourself, obviously!—read, write in a journal, or call a friend or family member. We also find that we often wake up in a state of what I call "ketone clarity" on the morning of a fast. This is the time we write down some of our best ideas, including the framework for this book. That said, while you might feel inspired to come up with a *Jerry Maguire* manifesto, we suggest you keep it to yourself rather than sending it to your boss. He or she might not share your feeling of enlightenment, and you don't want to end up getting fired like Jerry does in the movie. ("Who's coming with me?")

Another thing you can do here is to enhance the feeling of gratitude that we set in motion during the Vacation Night. While you're thinking or journaling, write a list of the top three things you're thankful for. The bed you slept in, your family, your hobbies. You could even go further and write down all the things you're thankful for, no matter how small they might seem. You may also find it useful to start thinking back over what you've achieved in recent weeks and how these positive actions have advanced your goals, whether that's in your career, education, personal life, or any other area.

We also challenge you to look to the future. Sure, this can mean jotting down some things you've got to get done later today or by the end of the week. But beyond this, we'd like you to set a big goal for yourself. Again, this can be work- or school-related, but it doesn't have to be. Just put down an ambitious aim that you want to shoot for and that's going to take a while to achieve, whether that's a few months, a year, or longer. As renowned author and speaker Greg Reid once said, "A dream written down with a date becomes a goal. A goal broken down into steps becomes a plan. A plan backed by action makes your dreams come true."

Your dream should be something that, while achievable, seems very ambitious and has a pretty high degree of difficulty. Maybe it's going back to school to finish that course you dropped out of or going one step further and getting your master's degree or a doctorate. Or it might be a fitness-related goal, such as doing a marathon or finishing an obstacle race. Perhaps it's not just about you but advances something you started during the Vacation Night, like spending more time with your kids each evening. The fact that you picked up this book and bought it shows that you have aspirations, and as you've gotten this far in the fast, you also possess the fortitude to turn a dream into reality.

Once you've named the goal (no matter how lofty it might seem), next write down an action plan. What's it going to take to get you to where you want to be? Write down a few smaller milestones that you're going to need to hit before reaching your ultimate destination. If dates are relevant, pull out a calendar and write the stepping-stone goals in your journal or notebook. Now we want you to execute. The best-laid plans are useless without action. So decide on the first step you need to take and implement it. As Yoda says in *Star Wars*, "Do or do not. There is no try."

YOUR GOAL & ACTION PLAN

Write three goals:

1. _____

2. _____

3. _____

Circle one goal.

Action plan: _____

_____

Execute that plan.

EXAMPLE

Write three goals:

1. Improve a relationship

2. Run a 5K

3. Go back to college

Action plan: If you circled #2, an example of an action plan might be: Go buy running shoes/clothes, pick a race in three to six months, tell friends that you're running the race (accountability), and find a web-based or personal training program.

Execute: Go out for a run.

REWIRING THE REWARD MECHANISM

The good news is that we have ways of helping you stay strong and resist the temptation to raid the fridge or pantry. We need to recognize that ghrelin, one of the hormones that promotes hunger, is going to be higher now than during the Vacation Night or ketotic sleep phases of the fast. The impulse that it urges us to fulfill—eat!—not only involves the digestive system but also areas of the brain like the nucleus accumbens. This is the reward center of the brain, which lights up when we complete the kind of habit loop Charles Duhigg describes in *The Power of Habit* with a pleasurable reward. As we know from earlier in the book, one of the main ways we like to trigger this and the accompanying flow of feel-good chemicals is through food. But that's not an option, at least for another few hours. So we need to build an alternative reward system.

Drinking plenty of high-quality water is not only for hydration but has an added benefit of a reward in that it continues the "oral fixation" habit that other food and drinks usually occupy. During this morning, have an ever-present glass of cold water near you and enjoy often.

If you didn't get a massage during the first part of the fast, we think you'll agree that it's even better when you've been running on ketones for a bit longer. If you're an avid exerciser, you can also do your workout as normal (see the Fasting for High Performance chapter for further guidance). Without going on and on, take a moment to list five alternate rewards for you:

1. _____

2. _____

3. _____

4. _____

5. _____

Is caffeine in your daily routine or listed as a reward above? While it is a mild stimulant of the central nervous system, caffeine also has the transient benefit of suppressing our appetite. As we are removing the "food" reward this morning, we don't wish to remove the "caffeine" reward as well. So if you're a coffee or tea drinker, we urge you to avoid going cold turkey on the caffeine. But as we are trying to help you de-stress and calm your body down, we advise tapering to 50 to 75 percent of your normal intake. The goal is to equalize the elevated effect caffeine may have on an empty stomach. This can mean reducing the amount or, if you like to sip a whole mug over the course of a morning, tapering down the caffeine with a "half-caff" blend. Take time to enjoy not only the taste of your beverage but also the warmth of the cup in your hands. This is another opportunity to be present, thankful, and aware. Try to avoid milk, creamer, sugar, or syrup, as these will technically break your fast.

While we're more than OK with you drinking tea or coffee, we suggest that you avoid drinking so-called energy drinks during this Spa Morning. The quantities of caffeine in such beverages can be far more than anything you'd find at your local coffee shop—unless you're pounding 10-shot Americanos throughout the day. In addition, many manufacturers add other chemical stimulants designed to amplify the effects of the caffeine. Then there's the high quantity of added sugar in a lot of these drinks that will break your fast if you drink a can.

UNPLUGGING FROM THE FOOD MATRIX

Another tactic to help this final phase of the fast be pleasant is to take your mind off of food, literally. One way to do this is to stay out of your refrigerator and pantry. We also suggest avoiding walking by your favorite restaurant or bakery as the wafting smell of breakfast or freshly baked bread might be too much to resist. In addition, you could extend your technology fast from the Vacation Night. By not watching TV, turning on your tablet, or opening your laptop lid, you're ensuring that you avoid food-related ads. This is only one type of mind control that you would do well to consciously avoid during the Spa Morning. Any kind of advertising is going to perpetuate a "more is more" commercialism mindset that runs counter to the "less is more" resetting practices we're discussing in this chapter.

LET LIFE UNFOLD

One way to accomplish calm during the morning phase of your fast is to clear your schedule. Make a deliberate effort to set aside 30 minutes to focus on nothing else but your own thoughts. If you have a spouse, kids, or housemates, this might seem impossible due to the other people in your living space. That's even more reason to wake up 30 minutes—and eventually 45 minutes or an hour—earlier than usual. This way you'll get in some "me time" before you start focusing on the needs of others. And don't worry, there will be plenty to do on that front later in this Spa Morning.

Let's check back in with Sam George on this topic. "We get so fixated on filling every day with as much activity as possible that we crowd out space to contemplate, reflect, and be," Sam said. "If we can build some gaps back in, we stop trying to force our will on outcomes and begin allowing life to unfold. And when you achieve stillness of thought by making time for it, all kinds of interesting things can happen."[49]

ACTIVITIES AND EXERCISE

Practices used during *The 17 Hour Fast* may also be incorporated into non-fast days and everyday life. Other beneficial activities include more mobility work to relieve tension from tight tissues and low-intensity workouts like yoga or Pilates. Or you could take a nice warm bath or soak in a hot tub. If you're going to get a massage or self-mobilize, many find it beneficial to prepare their bodies by performing a set of bodyweight exercises like push-ups, pull-ups, air squats, and lunges, incorporating as much of the body as possible. Doing these kinds of exercises for 20 to 25 minutes serves to potentiate the massage by increasing circulation and body temperature while also increasing muscle and tendon pliability and joint mobility.

For your first *17 Hour Fast*, we suggest that you stick with light exercise as your body is trying to figure out how to handle the new experience of abstaining from food. But once you have progressed from being a fasting rookie and have a few weeks of successful fasts under your belt, you can begin to dial up the intensity level. Our friend Brian Mackenzie, co-author of the book *Unplugged*, routinely gets up, walks his dogs, performs his breathing exercises, and goes to Jiu-Jitsu practice for two to three hours before breaking his fast.

Our VitalityPro camps are performed during *The 17 Hour Fast* and include a myriad of engineered modalities. You're welcome to join us at a camp and can find upcoming dates at www.myvitalitypro.com.

HARNESSING THE "HUNGER" MINDSET

Though I'm blessed to have a job which allows me to add value to people's lives and have found additional purpose in fulfilling my promise to Jason, I don't want to feel totally full and satisfied either. Instead, I want to retain that "hunger" I felt growing up in modest circumstances in small-town Alabama. Whether that was the desire to excel in athletics or the way I challenged myself while at the University of Alabama School of Medicine, I developed a hunger to push for more.

Brandon credits *The 17 Hour Fast* with giving him a "hungry" mindset when he starts the Spa Morning or, more often than not, when he's fasting at a VitalityPro camp where he's exerting himself and encouraging our athletes, first responders, and other attendees to do the same. "I like waking up hungry to get after the day ahead," he said. "If I wake up with a little physical hunger, that reminds me of the mindset I should approach the camp with—determined, wanting more. Now that I've been doing the fast for a couple of years, I know that my body will take care of that food-related hunger by fueling itself, while I focus on coaching and helping others."[50]

BRING ON ADVERSITY

We do just about everything we can to make our lives as comfortable as possible, which means avoiding adversity because we think it's unpleasant. But name one thing in your life that is worthwhile and *hasn't* required confronting and overcoming some level of difficulty? Try to come up with a single memorable achievement from your past that didn't cost you something. We bet you'll draw a blank on both fronts. Marriage, friendships, and a career all take substantial time and effort and require us to overcome problems and setbacks.

In medical school, I had plenty of classmates who were smarter and more talented than me. Some of them were second, third, or fourth generation doctors with a proud family tradition of practicing medicine. But anytime I was feeling intimidated by them or down on myself, my mom would remind me, "Nobody can outwork you." So I stuck with it, defied the odds, and graduated. That's not because I'm so great, but rather because I knuckled down and worked hard to make the most of the opportunity. Speaking of medical school, a young family friend who is about to graduate asked me whether he should do his residency at this state-of-the-art facility in a rich part of town or at an old, outdated community hospital in the rough inner city. I told him that in terms of real-world experience, there was no comparison—go with the inner city hospital because overcoming the challenges you'll face there will make you a better doctor and a better person.

We also need to relearn the lesson that it's not good to give into gratification each and every time we feel like we want something. The world of one-click online shopping and on-demand TV has offered us the false impression that we can and should have everything we want right now. But giving into this mindset is profoundly dangerous and, while we might not like to admit it, very unsatisfying. As German psychologist Erich Fromm put it, "Unrestricted satisfaction of all desires is not conducive to wellbeing, nor is it the way to happiness." And in fact, reckless indulgence can lead to misery. Phil's wife, Nicole, used to work for a bankruptcy attorney and came up with plans to help people have more self-discipline in their spending. We believe that the simple act of fasting once a week can help you develop discipline, which can then be directed into other aspects of your life. It can be a "want" reset button, if you will.

Which brings us back to this stage of the fast. While we hope we're helping you create a largely pleasant experience that you'll want to come back to and try again next week, you might well confront some challenges. Maybe it's the habitual temptation to grab a snack from your pantry. Perhaps it's some hunger pains that start gnawing at you. Or it could be that you begin feeling a bit physically weak, right as a little voice in your head starts telling you that you can't finish the fast. We've had to work through all of these things and more. And we can tell you from personal experience the sense of accomplishment we've felt, knowing that we remained resolute until the end. The great thing about *The 17 Hour Fast* is that each time you do it, it becomes a bit easier. But first, you need to face that adversity head on, harness your hunger, and let this drive you toward success. Tell yourself that completing the fast is your only option, and do what it takes to win. You'll be so glad you did.

THE 17 HOUR FAST FOR THE WORKER

If you have to work the morning of your fast, you might not be able to ease into the day or use all the practices we're talking about in this chapter. Yet many of the concepts can still be used if slightly modified. What I've found to be helpful on days that I'm fasting and working in the ER is to wake up even earlier than when I'm fasting on my days off. This way I'm not making myself frantic before I even get out the door. In fact, I do everything I can to set my day up for tranquility. I'll have a cool glass of water and then a little coffee before carving out a few minutes for thought, prayer, and meditation. Then I'll leave the house a few minutes earlier than I really need to. That way I won't be stressed out if there's a wreck or roadwork blocking my way to the hospital. When I get to the ER, I try to make sure I'm doing things a little more steadily and deliberately than usual, in an attempt to project a sense of calm to my colleagues and patients from the get go. Trust me, the day will have enough stress and I don't need to add to it. I'm sure your day has its pressures too, and an early rise can help you deal with them better.

When we initially started doing *The 17 Hour Fast*, we used Spa Morning rewards to make the process more enjoyable and to build a positive mental association with fasting. As we continued fasting weekly, the mere act of doing the fast became its own reward. Now many of us fast to make working, traveling for business, and so on more pleasurable.

THE CALORIE AND GOODWILL EXCHANGE CHALLENGE

Earlier we heard from Coach Gene Stallings about how he would sit down to a family dinner with his wife and children and put work aside during that time. Now let's discover what he did in between leaving the University of Alabama campus and getting home. "After practice, I stopped by the hospital practically every night," Coach Stallings said. "There was always someone who was sick and whose family would ask me to visit them, so I'd go sit with kids, older folks, and Alabama fans of all ages."[51] When we asked him how he managed to devote daily time to helping others while running a national, championship-winning football program, Coach Stallings simply said, "You just have to fit it into your schedule."[52] So while random acts of kindness and impromptu generosity are both good things, scheduling service to others is a way to make sure it doesn't get crowded out. Whether it's during your Spa Mornings or on other days throughout the week, let's block off time for giving and volunteering.

Up until this point, we've mainly talked about focusing on you during this Spa Morning. Now we're going to shift the focus onto other people. As the obesity stats show that millions of us in this country are having problems handling an abundance of food, there are plenty of folks who have the opposite issue. They're not just waking up a little hungry one day a week but starting each and every day feeling famished. While many of us need to let go of a few calories if we're to have longer and higher quality lives, they're desperately seeking a way to get more calories just so they can survive and have any kind of life. Interesting, isn't it? Data actually supports that for us and them both to live better and longer, they literally need to eat some of our calories. This isn't just a challenge that affects those in the developing world, though their needs are extremely pressing. There are people in your state, your city, and maybe even your community who have an urgent need to eat more.

Even though it appears that we have shifted the focus from you to others, remember you'll reap many rewards from helping them. A team led by Dr. Suzanne Richards at the University of Exeter Medical School reviewed 40 studies from the past 20 years on the link between volunteering and health. The article, which is freely available in the open-access journal BMC Public Health, finds that volunteering is associated with lower depression, increased well-being, and a 22 percent reduction in the risk of dying.[53] Whether you're giving actual food, money for food, or an act of kindness and goodwill, everybody wins.

During the Vacation Night, we evaluated how we spend our time to honestly appraise how we're either nurturing or neglecting our relationships and to use that time to start reordering our calendar priorities. Well, now we'd like to take a look at checking accounts and credit card statements and see how much of a priority giving is in your life. This simple exercise isn't intended to guilt us into giving more but rather should prompt a candid assessment of where we're directing our funds, which also goes a long way to revealing our true priorities. If we're regularly setting aside some money for a cause we're passionate about, then great. If not, perhaps this is a good time to start.

Earlier we talked about setting goals, writing out an action plan, and taking the first step toward achieving it. Now we want to be similarly proactive on behalf of someone else. The challenge with hunger is that it seems too big for us. How can we possibly feed the millions of people around the world who are malnourished? We can when we take the "I'm one person and I *can* help one person" attitude.

We all wrestle with compassion fatigue. When we see a news story on a famine in an African nation or get yet another food bank flyer in the mail, it's tempting to switch off our empathy for others and look the other way. But whether you believe in God or not, we'd urge you to do as the Bible says in the book of Galatians and "never tire of doing good." Compassion fatigue is a cop-out enabled by our state of perpetual distraction. What we fail to realize is that while the issue of hunger might not directly affect our family, it's impacting somebody who has parents, siblings, kids, and grandkids just like we do. Someone who feels pain and anguish every day. And someone who can benefit directly from our kindness and generosity. That's why we're asking you to give during your Spa Morning.

Robert Louis Stevenson once said, "Don't judge each day by the harvest you reap but by the seeds that you plant." You've already rewarded yourself, and now it's time to reward someone else. Plant those seeds. Mac Powell told us that when we fast:

> "We can get beyond the physical needs we're usually so fixated on, and start thinking about other areas of our lives. Then we can begin to get outside ourselves and consider the needs of others and what we can do to help meet these. I remember that at the end of *Schindler's List*, the guy is looking at his gold wedding ring and regrets not selling it because that could've saved a few more lives. That's a powerful image of what it means to really give and then think about how we can give some more. We all have different ways to do that. I've got a platform to reach a big audience with my voice. For someone else, it might be serving at a homeless shelter. Awards and other accolades quickly fade away. It's the impact that you make on other people that's really important."[54]

We're not talking about making a massive donation here, though if you have the means and the heart to do so, that would be fantastic. Whether it's giving to a charity like Food for the Hungry or World Vision online (yes, you get a technology hall pass to do it, but be sure to shut your laptop lid when you're done), mailing a check to an organization like Harvesters or Feeding America, or contributing to an inner city school's backpack lunch program, you can make a meaningful difference in a life right now. Another more hands-on way to help is to take some cans and dry goods to your local food bank.

To further encourage your giving, we have a page on our website dedicated to this, the Calorie and Goodwill Exchange, which you can find listed under Charities at www.17hourfast.com. There, you'll see a broad range of non-profits like the ones we've featured at the end of this chapter and those supported by the people we interviewed. Please consider giving to one of these or an organization that you're fond of, knowing that we're doing the same by giving 10 percent of our royalties to these great, life-changing causes. And by purchasing this book, you're helping us make a greater contribution.

This initiative isn't merely about money. You could give your time as well, such as by volunteering to serve lunch at a local soup kitchen or packing food for Backpacks for Kids. I've done the latter many times, along with Regina and the boys. There's something so moving about looking into the eyes of a fellow human and seeing the gratitude when you put a simple meal in their hands. It's also very humbling to witness how much of a struggle some people have just to meet this basic need. We believe it sets our children up well to understand just how blessed they are and how they can make a positive difference in our community by simply giving an hour or two of their time every week.

One of the people our family looks to for an example of selflessness is Jesse Billauer. Back in the mid-90s, Jesse was ranked in the top 100 junior surfers on the planet and was about to turn pro. But on a fateful Malibu morning in March 1996, a wave viciously threw him down into a sandbar, breaking his sixth vertebrae. Jesse's dream of a long and decorated surfing career was over, and in an instant, this vigorous young man became a quadriplegic.

Such an incident would crush the spirit of many people. But as he lay in his hospital bed, he started dreaming another dream—one that would see him getting back on his board and helping others with physical challenges do the same. That vision blossomed into what is now the non-profit Life Rolls On, which not only provides surfing-based experiences for young people but also exposes them to skateboarding. As for Jesse, he overcame the longest of odds and became a champion. He shared with us how he used something that could easily be seen as bad for the good of others:

"A lot of people look at those like me who are in wheelchairs and think we can't do a lot. Sometimes we start to believe it too or get so scared of the unknown that we won't try something new. Getting out in the water or on a skateboard gives us back a sense of freedom and independence.

YOUR CHARITABLE GOAL & ACTION PLAN

Write three charitable goals:

1. _____

2. _____

3. _____

Circle one goal.

Action plan: _____

_____

Execute that plan.

EXAMPLE

Write three charitable goals:

1. Donate $15 I would have spent on breakfast to Food for the Hungry at www.fh.org

2. Help serve food at local homeless shelter

3. Pack Backpacks for Kids for local school

Action plan: If you circled #1, log on briefly and donate.

Execute: Donate that $15 or completely support a child for just a little more money. Now take a "Genesis breath" and feel good about what you just did for someone in need.

You only need to look at the huge smiles on kids' faces to see the impact it's having on them. They might have felt shy or left out at school, but many parents have told me that they go back with a new sense of confidence and start making friends who also surf or skate. We've had people who meet at our events and eventually get married. It's helping build new relationships and a sense of community. When people get the chance to know each other better, it makes the world smaller and brings us closer together. I just wanted to do my part to help a few people in my community, and it's grown into something more."[55]

We asked Jesse when and where he had learned to be charitable and focus on others. He revealed that it was a natural emotion and reaction that developed within him during the initial days after the accident. We're amazed that his intuition and instinct alone guided him to do what many studies reveal—that individuals have more personal success when they focus on helping others.

Whatever way you choose to be inspired by Jesse's example to help others, thank you so much for your generosity of spirit and action. As Mac Powell told us recently, "You don't have to do everything to help others, but you should do something."[56]

List of Charities Suggested/Supported by Our Contributors and Us

Gene Stallings: RISE Program, Live Beyond
Jeremiah Castille: Jeremiah Castille Foundation
Jesse Billauer: Life Rolls On
Mac Powell: Food for the Hungry
Peter Furler: ChildFund International
Randy Rarick: Surfing Heritage Foundation

Others

Food for the Poor
Catholic Relief Services
Children's Hunger Fund
Samaritan's Purse
Compassion International

Nick's Kids
Kidz1stFund
Tim Tebow Foundation
Feed God's Hungry Children
Aid for Starving Children
Americans Helping Americans
The Water Project
A Mission for Children
Children's Feeding Network
Salvation Army
Operation Blessing International
Panama City Rescue Mission
Rainbow Omega
Anchorage Children's Home
St. Andrew Community Medical Center
Feeding America
The Hunger Project
Backpack Blessings
Living Water International
Angel Flight
Surfrider Foundation
SurfAid
Made in the Streets
Operation Smile
St. Jude Children's Research Hospital
Wounded Warrior Project
Lt. Michael P. Murphy Memorial Scholarship Foundation
Operation Second Chance
Pat Tillman Foundation
Global Citizen Foundation
The Last Well

POST-FAST MEALS

Now that we've explored each phase of the fast itself—the pre-fast meals, Vacation Night, ketotic sleep, and Spa Morning—it's time to move onto what you do afterward. Even though it's tempting to think that you're done now that you can eat again, the book isn't over. One of the ways that we extend the benefits of *The 17 Hour Fast* and start reaping some of the rewards of a longer one is to approach our first post-fast meal deliberately and carefully. Remember that each stage of this protocol has been painstakingly formulated to give us maximum benefit.

So before you rush headlong into a super-sized lunch in the mistaken belief that you need to make up for not eating for 17 hours, we encourage you to read this chapter thoughtfully with the same sense of self-control and purpose as you just applied to the previous phases. If you do, you'll find that the fast has a far greater positive impact than if you simply loaded up a big plate and went to town. You've made a significant effort to retool your eating habits and lifestyle practices, and it makes no sense to undo most or all of your good work by giving in to overindulgence now.

Before we jump into the nitty gritty of the post-fast meal, we first want to say congratulations. You've completed your first *17 Hour Fast*! This might seem like a small thing, but it's not. Whether you were skeptical about fasting or jumped in wholeheartedly with both feet, you did something highly meaningful and purposeful. If you've had a dysfunctional relationship with food for years or even decades, you just took a big first step in putting things back in perspective. In addition, you completed the most important training session you'll ever do—one that started reconditioning your liver and pancreas.

At the same time, you gave your overworked digestive system the rest it has been craving for so long. And speaking of craving, you proved to yourself that you're strong enough to resist the temptation to snack all day and night. Plus, you were able to prioritize restoration through a restful evening and retooled your sleep hygiene to deliver premium, reparative slumber. You also made a commitment to better protect your experiences with family and friends, to set up stronger boundaries around work and technology, and carved out some truly high quality time to help yourself and, more importantly, other people.

Now let's rejoice and refuel. You should feel proud that you set a goal, followed the steps needed to achieve it, and then finished the job. Don't dismiss your accomplishment because it matters more than you understand. Now you know that you've done the fast once, believe that you can build on this and commit to repeating it once a week. We'll get to some tricks and tips for making the experience even better and amplifying the benefits in a little bit, but first let's take care of your most pressing need: food! Eventually, you might get to the point where you feel so good at the end of the 17 hours that you don't want to eat right away, but that isn't typical with first timers.

PLAYING THE PERCENTAGES

We recommend that your post-fast lunch and dinner look a lot like your pre-fast lunch and dinner. Aim for about 75 percent of your usual calorie and portion size, and try to keep your carbs to 20 percent of total calories at lunch and 30 percent at dinner. Note that these percentages are your end goals as you perfect the fast and therefore may be less attainable and unwise for the initial fasts. Example: if your normal meal is say 60 percent carbs, you may wish to try a 10 percent reduction per fast or per month to an ending goal of 20 percent at lunch and 30 percent at supper. Remember, it's the tortoise and the hare. It's important to be cognizant of the fact that carbs vary in how quickly and to what extent they impact your blood sugar levels. Remember from chapter 4 that many carb-rich foods are composed of fast-acting sugars that send your blood sugar through the roof and then bring you back down with a crash. We suggest that you limit these foods (including candy, desserts, and certain fruits) or exclude them entirely—the glycemic index chart that we referred to earlier, which shows how much a food raises your blood sugar, will give you a good idea of which foods to avoid. Instead, opt for healthy, slow-digesting carbs that won't spike your blood sugar like leafy green vegetables, root vegetables like sweet potatoes and carrots, squash, and tomatoes. You can also include whole grains, such as oats, brown rice, and quinoa (the latter packs a hefty protein punch as well).

When it comes to carbs, it's not just what you eat that you need to consider. Many people unwittingly take in a lot of sugar in juices, blended coffee drinks, and the like. If you exercised, it's OK to have a little chocolate milk (go with an organic option with minimal sugar) to replenish glycogen levels or a very small glass of fruit juice that doesn't have any added sugar. But drinking a liter of either isn't the way ahead. If you're going to have coffee, stick to the black stuff itself or coffee with milk and stay away from the sugar packets and syrups. Prefer tea? Then also avoid putting in any sweeteners unless it's a dash of local raw honey.

For the post-fast lunch, ensure 40 percent of the calories come from good fats like those found in avocados, olive oil, nuts, and a little full-fat, organic dairy. Then use lean meats or fish for the protein (forty percent of total calories). My favorite post-fast lunch is usually in the hospital cafeteria. I typically choose a big salad with lettuce, spinach, arugula, and other greens, some peppers, chopped carrots, and whatever veggies they're offering that day. I throw in a couple of ounces of steak, chicken, or turkey and add in some olive oil and a little balsamic vinegar. The post-fast dinner is 35 percent fat and protein and up to 30 percent low-glycemic-index carbohydrates.

Dialing in your post-fast meals should be about pursuing continual improvement. It's also a good idea to try and mirror the approach you took with your pre-fast lunch and dinner—in terms of portion size and protein/fat/carbs breakdown—as closely as possible so you get some of the ketogenesis-related benefits for your liver, pancreas, digestive system, mood, and cellular biology that you usually only find with a longer fast of 24, 36, 48, or 72 hours (while avoiding their potential pitfalls). One of these benefits is continuing to provide a slightly more optimal blend of

PUT IN SOME PREBIOTICS

Probiotics are all the rage, and while these can be beneficial, you shouldn't forget about prebiotics, which can aid digestion, help improve the diversity of your gut flora, and encourage the activity of health-promoting bacteria. The good news is they are found naturally in foods like bananas, asparagus, artichokes (particularly the Jerusalem variety), leeks, onions, and garlic, which you can easily add to your post-fast meals and throughout the week. Your gut will thank you!

glucose and ketones and getting every cell in your body more efficient with using this new flex fuel cocktail. Creating some degree of symmetry between your pre- and post-fast meals will also mean you're not shocking your system with a massive calorie surplus or deficit or an unexpected and unfamiliar balance of macro and micronutrients.

PRECISION MATTERS

The micronutrient breakdowns in this chapter and for your pre-fast meals might seem a little persnickety. But realize that the margin between success and failure really is razor-thin. For example, we worked with a triple jumper who was trying to qualify for the 2016 Rio Olympics. On his final attempt at the Olympic trials, he sailed down that runway, soared through the air, and leaped his way to a qualifying distance. There was just one very small problem. His shoe had indented the soft clay takeoff strip by a couple of millimeters. Even though this seems like a minor infraction, it was enough for the judge to rule his effort a "no jump." Despite jumping further than most of the field, he had fallen agonizingly short of his bid to make the team and would have to commit to four years of training to have another shot.

We apply a similar, measured, highly detailed approach to each and every stage of *The 17 Hour Fast*. Like the qualifying distances and times for Olympians (not to mention that big rule book), we use very precise calculations

THE POST-FAST LUNCH AND DINNER BREAKDOWNS

Here are the macronutrient percentages and portion sizes we recommend for your two post-fast meals. See chapter 11 for tips on changing your macronutrient breakdowns incrementally over time. If you're an athlete, please disregard these numbers in favor of those in the next chapter.

POST-FAST LUNCH

Fats: 40 percent   *Protein:* 40 percent   *Carbs:* 20 percent
Portion size/calories: 75 percent of your usual lunch.
If you're trying to lose weight, aim for 50 percent.

POST-FAST DINNER

Fats: 35 percent   *Protein:* 35 percent   *Carbs:* 30 percent
Portion size/calories: 75 percent of your usual dinner if you're at a healthy
BMI/body fat percentage/weight. If you're trying to lose weight,
try to stick with this reduced calorie/portion (75 percent)
each subsequent meal for as long as you can into the rest of the week.

that we've tinkered with for many years to perfect. We've not only gone deep into inter-disciplinary research and consulted with experts in many specialties, but we have also relentlessly field tested our protocols with a broad range of people, from first responders and members of the armed forces to elite athletes to everyday folks like you and me. So while this isn't a one-size-fits-all plan—and we want you to become your own experiment and play with the percentages—know that we have put thousands of hours into coming up with the details for your post-fast meals.

BREAKING YOUR FAST THE RIGHT WAY

When you fast, your body flushes out bad bacterial overgrowth and sometimes undigested or semi-digested pieces of food that might be interfering with normal digestive function. Earlier on in the Spa Morning chapter, we implored you to include drinking a big glass of cold water soon after you wake and frequently thereafter to avoid dehydration during the fast. This will also assist the spring cleaning process in the gut. Before you begin eating the post-fast lunch, we encourage you to "prime the pump" with a glass or two of cool water, which will aid in anatomical satiety, helping you to not overeat.

When it comes to the post-fast lunch, I'm not going to claim that I'm blameless when it comes to nutrition. So I'll admit to you that sometimes I'll sprinkle a tablespoon or so of Craisins into my salad bowl. Yes, yes, I know they're super high in sugar. But I believe that we can't be perfect all the time and need a little something we know isn't so great for us to go along with a lot of what is. When I eat my big salad, I usually just drink water.

As you haven't eaten in a little while and your stomach should be fully empty, your digestive system is going to be primed to prioritize the first thing you send to it after breaking your fast. So try to make sure it's something beneficial and worthwhile that your body can use for the good, like fat and protein (fish, steak, or turkey, or if you're vegetarian, tofu or beans) or micronutrient-rich veggies (kale, broccoli, and lettuce, for example), rather than a quick simple sugar hit that's going to send you right back to step one again. You've created a hunger-based demand, so now make sure the supply is just right. Otherwise you'll be putting low-grade gas in your Ferrari engine (we don't own supercars, but we're guessing that nobody who does is choosing 85-grade gas at the pump).

When we're doing a camp, something else we like to take in after breaking our fast is a kombucha drink that one of our partners, Finn's Restaurant, prepares for us. We'll alternate between this and one of our favorites from Ollo's in Malibu, a carrot/turmeric/ginger blend. It contains a couple of ounces of orange juice but not enough to spike blood-glucose levels. I've started adding a pinch of cayenne pepper as it has antimicrobial qualities and assists in flushing out overgrowth of bad gut bacteria. I also enjoy adding espresso back into my diet once I'm through fasting—though not with the kombucha drink, which would taste awful! Try to avoid pressuring yourself into cramming every good food into your first post-fast meal. If you've got a range of vegetables, fruits, healthy fats, and proteins in mind, split them between your post-fast lunch and dinner.

Speaking of that first post-fast dinner, we suggest mirroring what you did with your lunch if you're trying to lose weight and reduce your body fat percentage: keeping the portion/calorie intake to 75 percent of your usual meal and sticking with a ratio of 35 percent fat, 35 percent protein, and 30

150

WHAT IF YOU COULDN'T FINISH THE FAST?

We're confident that you got to 17 hours before breaking your fast. But we know plenty of people who haven't quite made it. Reasons include feeling a little woozy, like they have low energy, or that they just couldn't hold off their habitual eating habit any longer (and a whole host of others). If this is you this first time, don't be hard on yourself! It's sometimes a lot easier to give other people grace than ourselves. Even if you didn't get to 17 hours, we still want to say "well done" for a solid effort. Give yourself a pat on the back and resolve to try again next week.

There's no shame in doing a 16, 15, or 14 hour fast, and we sometimes do that ourselves. From a numbers standpoint, you still likely made it 70, 80, or 90 percent of the way, and on your first try too. And if you stick to the post-fast meal recommendations, those percentages will go up. That's very good going. If, say, you made it as far as 14 hours, go for 14 and a half next week, and then try adding 30 minutes a week thereafter until you hit 17. Maybe you'll find it easier to go the distance if you ask a family member or friend to fast with you. Even if you hit a wall and have to stay at 14, 15, or however many hours, you're still deriving many of the benefits of the full fast, not to mention the positive lifestyle changes that you're implementing along the way. So stop giving yourself a hard time and please stick with the fast.

percent non-refined carbs. In the following days, see how long you can keep your calorie intake at three fourths of your typical dinner total. Maybe you will eventually reduce this to 50 percent. This is easier in reality than it might sound because your body can change its baselines very quickly, and by doing the fast, you've already shifted the goalposts in a good way. If you can go for long enough, you'll not only start moving toward your weight/fat loss target but will also establish a new normal for what a typical meal looks like. As we wrote earlier, *The 17 Hour Fast* can have a positive ripple effect throughout your life, and this is just one example that our clients and friends have benefited from.

AVOIDING THE ON-THE-GO LUNCH TRAP

We hope that over the past 17 hours, you've fully embraced the concept of turning down the speed dial on your life so that you can enjoy each and every moment to the fullest. This includes the pace at which you eat. If you recall, we advised you back in the Pre-Fast Meals chapter to double the number of times you chew and enjoy each bite during your pre-fast lunch and dinner. We'd like you to continue this now that you're breaking the fast. It's tempting to look at the Vacation Night and Spa Morning through a productivity lens and see a big waste of task-completing time. Doing so will likely spur you to rush through this post-fast lunch so you can get to all the stuff you didn't do this morning and yesterday evening.

Don't do it! Instead, take your time and enjoy this first meal of the day. During the pro surfing tour season, Randy Rarick meets sponsors for lavish dinners every night and knows that by the time the final event of the Triple Crown is over, he's right into the overindulgence of Christmas meals with family and friends, which we can certainly relate to. So by the time he gets to the New Year, Randy takes deliberate measures to reset his baseline:

> "In January, I stop drinking completely, consume smaller portions and try to eat more vegetables and salads. This helps me lose a little of the weight I'd put on the previous few weeks, and I feel much better after four weeks of dialing things back a little. It also makes me appreciate that first glass of wine and the flavor of that first steak once I get into February."[57]

Follow Randy's lead and make an effort to enjoy your post-fast lunch. If you're at home, prepare a meal of fresh ingredients and either enjoy a little more me time or celebrate your successful fast with your family. Or if you're going to be eating out, then choose a restaurant with a calm environment rather than the hectic confines of a fast food joint, where the workers are moving at warp speed to satisfy the food-now demands of their hurrying customers. And don't just grab a sandwich and take it to your desk so that you can get back to work. Remember what we discussed about focusing on one thing at a time and becoming fully immersed in and aware of it? Instead of taking a hurried half-lunch at your desk, invite a friend or colleague to join you, and leave your phone turned off so you can enjoy their company and your conversation. If you must be at the office, at least go to the cafeteria or break room so you're not blurring the lines between a mealtime and work.

Savor your food, and don't be in a big rush to get to your next appointment. Earlier we touched on the idea of compressing or expanding time. Here's another example of how our over-enthusiastic scheduling can set us up for either a stressful day or a relaxing lunch. Create a midday gap so that you can be unhurried with this lunch. In turn, this will mean that your afternoon is less stressful and frenetic than usual. Realize that you can never get everything done in one day, and try to carry the steady pace of your morning over into this post-fast phase.

Looking beyond the post meal itself and the afternoon activities that follow, we also hope that some of the routines you started cultivating during your Vacation Night and Spa Morning will carry into this evening and tomorrow. Sure, you might need to play catch up from the fast, and your obligations and commitments aren't suddenly going to disappear. But we believe that by being more deliberate in how you approach the time that you dedicate to friends, family, and yourself, you'll be able to apply more structure to your work and extracurricular activities as well. And if you can start to better compartmentalize your day, you will probably be more productive, less reactive, and less frazzled than before you started fasting.

FASTING *for* HIGH PERFORMANCE

We've thoroughly explored the various stages of *The 17 Hour Fast,* from the pre-fast meals all the way through the post-fast meals. Now it's time to look at how it can help athletes and high performers in the workplace meet their goals, excel at the highest level, and buffer extreme levels of stress. If you're one of these people, perhaps you've skipped to here from the introduction.

We can't blame you for doing so, as we often jump ahead in a book to the sections we think will be most beneficial. But once you're finished with this section, we implore you to rewind and read the preceding chapters as you'll find some tips and tricks that you can add to what you're about to discover in the following pages. Whichever way you ended up in this chapter, you're going to find out how to tweak *The 17 Hour Fast* to meet your performance and recovery demands, why it's perfect for dealing with the stressors and anxieties you face daily, and how it can help improve your relationships.

Our approach throughout this book is to create positive change in all aspects of your life, including body, mind, and soul. Let's look at the body first.

PART I: BODY

Training Your Liver and Pancreas

You spend so much time working on various elements of training to condition your muscles, connective tissues, heart, brain, and so on. So why would you let your fuel system (i.e., the liver and pancreas) become so deconditioned, inefficient, and ineffective at producing ketones or sourcing glucose from anything other than simple sugars? So many athletes have fine-tuned most of their preparation but left some low-hanging fruit—like training their liver and pancreas—on the tree. If you put two athletes with virtually the same physical capabilities and size next to each other, the one who can more effectively and efficiently fuel via both gluconeogenesis and ketogenesis in addition to carbohydrate digestion will have a natural advantage.

This is not only because they can tap into the longer-lasting fuel of ketones and are better at using certain amino acids to make glucose, but also because every cell in their body is better at using both of these fuel types to power performance. And the best part about it is that they can get such an advantage naturally, safely, and sustainably via the physiological adaptations and advancements that *The 17 Hour Fast* provides.

More on the Ketone/Glucose Blend Advantage

Eating poorly is one of the biggest things that athletes can do to sabotage themselves. If over-training/under-recovering is the number one challenge active people face, we contend that bad eating habits may be number two. Nowhere is this truer than in the endurance sports community. For decades, runners, swimmers, cyclists, rowers, and so on have maintained their energy levels by refueling every 20, 30, or 45 minutes. This fuel often comes in the form of so-called "sports drinks," gels, tabs, and such, the ingredients of which include simple sugars and electrolytes.

The trouble is that by constantly topping off the body's fuel tank, we make ourselves believe that we're a car that can only go two miles before stopping at the gas station again. Even if you're nowhere close to a hypermiler, would you buy a car that only got two miles to the gallon? Of course not! But the way we approach nutrition as athletes is the equivalent of that gas guzzler. Our bodies were designed to be like a Prius, a Tesla, or one of those tiny, super-efficient, clean diesel cars you see zipping around London or Paris.

We should be able to go for hundreds of miles on a tank of gas and be so efficient at using every drop of fuel we put in that we're getting 60 mpg.

But when we're constantly topping off the tank with refined sugars, we can lose some ability to produce ketones from fat and two amino acids (leucine and lysine).

Now if you're reading this as an athlete who has been conditioned to believe you need a sports drink, bar, or gel every 20 to 30 minutes so you don't "bonk," you might be thinking, "I can't afford to have even a 3 percent decrease in my performance due to a drop in blood-glucose levels." But in reality, if you're training or performing while taking in sugars, you may be losing more than 3 percent performance by diverting blood supply from your muscles, heart, lungs, and brain to your digestive system to metabolize that sugar. So if you were able to keep, say, 10 percent performance advantage by keeping blood flow directed to muscles and vital organs involved in the game and lose the theoretical 3 percent advantage of the glucose, you would still have a net gain of 7 percent performance advantage. That's a big deal, particularly when we're thinking about the razor-thin margins at the highest level. Additionally, training- or event-related sugar intake can potentially produce other performance disadvantages, including turning on the parasympathetic nervous system, reactive hypoglycemia (the "bonk"), indigestion, diarrhea, and dehydration. Please understand that we encourage replacement of water and electrolytes.

We also believe that some of the supposed benefit of keeping blood sugar topped up is mostly a placebo effect. It provides comfort because you believe that you perform better when you're constantly taking in simple carbs. Many of the issues people deal with when exercising during their first few fasts are psychological too. They're expecting to feel like they are about to run out of energy or will fail to meet their usual standards, and this can become a self-fulfilling prophecy because the mind controls the body. Yet let's think about this logically for a moment. When you fast, you're not just training your body to produce more ketones, which deliver longer-lasting energy that doesn't wax and wane. You're also training your cells to better utilize this more stable fuel source. Plus, you're making your body more efficient at producing glucose and putting it to work. So it stands to reason that once your body gets used to the slightly different energy mixture coursing through it, you're going to be able to have better access to your metabolic potential for shorter, harder, more explosive activities and longer, slower endurance events alike.

Our biological imprint conditioned us to be able to store and utilize fat as fuel for all-day hunting and gathering. Our ancestors weren't running around with energy bars in their pockets or goos and gels in the pouches of their hydration vests. In fact, most of them didn't carry any food with them at all. Or if they did, it was the kind of high-fat, slow-metabolizing fuel that Chris McDougall's book *Born to Run* describes the Tarahumara tribe eating. (You know, those guys and girls who can run for hundreds of miles barefoot or in basic sandals through sweltering valleys in northern Mexico eating nothing more than chia seeds.)

The habits we've created to keep ourselves going are an artificial construct. We can either wait for our genetics and fundamental physiology to adapt to our new behavior or we can move forward by looking backward to how we were created to function and fuel—with larger, calorie-dense meals interspersed with periods of fasting.

Tweaking the Recipe

Almost every high performer you come across in any field—whether they are an athlete, work in a creative field, are an entrepreneur, or anything else—has a go-to routine. Some of them even stick with the same clothes, meals, and schedules because such consistency creates a sense of calm, reduces decision fatigue, and allows them to make controllable factors more predictable. Therefore, they have more capacity to deal with unforeseen problems and challenges. While it's great to have go-to habits and daily patterns, it can breed a sense of complacency and an unwillingness to change.

Such rigidity can prevent those who already have a successful track record from reaching even greater heights of achievement. This is a contrast to the world's best chefs, who are always tasting their signature recipes and tweaking the ingredients slightly to make their soups and stews even better. Like that master cook pulling back on the salt a little or adding a sprig of oregano, so too should the elite (or those who strive to be) in other professions seek to constantly be on the lookout for ways to improve their routines. One of the easiest life upgrades if you're in this category is to try *The 17 Hour Fast* and see what impact it has on your productivity, energy levels, and recovery.

POST-FAST MEAL BREAKDOWNS FOR MUSCLE GAIN

If you're an athlete who's trying to gain muscle, please disregard the post-fast meal breakdowns from earlier in the book and go with the following recommendations instead. Note that you should be splitting your post-fast lunch into two parts. This goes back to the concept we discussed earlier of driving demand with exercise and then supplying the nutrients needed to help you rebuild and recover—aka the "priming the pump" theory. Ingesting all your protein in a single-serving, post-workout lunch is not going to have the positive impact you hope for because your body will use a lot of that protein to make glucose and, to a lesser degree, ketones. That's why the protein shakes Brandon Rager and his college and NFL teammates used to drink after every morning practice didn't give them the recovery they wanted. You also don't want to shock your system by going from not eating for 17 hours to throwing down a massive lunch. Instead, you'll get all the nutrients your body needs to fuel muscle growth and repair at the right time with a staggered approach using the following protocol:

POST-FAST LUNCH PART ONE

Fat: 40 percent   *Protein:* 40 percent   *Carbs:* 20 percent
Calories: 75 to 100 percent of usual lunch

POST-FAST LUNCH PART TWO/SNACK (approx. two hours after lunch)

Fat: 10 percent   *Protein:* 70 percent   *Carbs:* 20 percent
Calories: 50 percent of usual lunch
(total of 125 to 150 percent when combined with post-fast lunch part one)

POST-FAST DINNER

Fat: 40 percent   *Protein:* 40 percent   *Carbs:* 20 percent
Calories: 100 to 125 percent of usual dinner
We recommend that you try to keep the 125 percent calorie intake going for
as many meals as possible to fuel muscle gain, as long as you keep training hard.

The Post-Workout Protein Deception

For years we've been told by magazines, blogs, and podcasts that we need to follow the "20-20" rule for post-workout refueling: getting 20 grams of complete protein within 20 minutes of a workout. If people are feeling really daring, they might advise that you change this to 30 grams within 30 minutes.

Now after you exercise, your body obviously needs to start the adaptation and repair process, and nutrition is a big part of this. But whether you're a high-level football player like Brandon was, a mid-level competitor, or just someone who likes to work out a few times a week, the old strategy of drinking a giant protein shake right away might not be the best plan.

There's also the fact that exercise is an appetite suppressant. That's why very few people are famished right after they practice or play a sport. It takes a while for the body to cycle down from a high level of exertion and start to prioritize recovery in a parasympathetic state instead of being on high alert and focusing on sustaining motion in a sympathetic mode. This is why for athletes who are trying to build muscle, we advocate splitting their post-exercise and post-fast lunch into two parts.

The first part features a greater percentage of carbs and fat than protein, which can meet your body's immediate energy needs. For this, we advise you choose some easily digestible plant sources like those found in beans, vegetables such as peas and broccoli, avocados, nuts, and seeds. If you want to have a smaller shake with some whey and berries, plus maybe some kind of nut butter, then you can do so, but make sure it's not a whole pitcher's worth. At VitalityPro camps, we usually have the following:

- 4 ounces kombucha
- A small "berry bowl" with a mix of various glycemic-index fruits, such as acai, strawberries, and blueberries
- Half an avocado with chipotle flakes and sea salt
- A hard-boiled egg
- About one square inch of dark chocolate
- A small cup of coffee

Then comes part two. About two to two-and-a-half hours after the first installment of your smaller post-fast lunch, it's time for a second serving. This time you're going to dial the protein up to 70 percent, as your body has topped off its glycogen stores with that first part of your lunch and will be better able to put protein to work for muscle building and repair. You can also go with slightly slower acting protein sources, like dairy products, fish, poultry, or beef. Sometimes we'll eat a small can of chicken or tuna and a piece of fruit. Again, this will be more of a snack-size portion. But if you're trying to maintain or

FINN'S BOWL, TOAST, AND OVERNIGHT OATS RECIPES

ACAI BOWL

Filtered water

Raw acai

Bananas

Blueberries

Strawberries

Agave nectar

BEES KNEES BOWL

Organic milk

Peanut butter

Bananas

Chia seeds

Peanuts

Honey

Bee pollen

BOOCH BOWL

Noli south

Kombucha

Blueberries

Strawberries

Chia seeds

Agave nectar

ENERGIZER BOWL

Coconut milk

Bananas

Protein powder

Cacao nibs

Chia seeds

Almonds

Almond butter

GREENS BOWL

Coconut water

Bananas

Mango

Pineapple

Protein powder

Spinach

Hemp seeds

Agave

UNDERTOW BOWL

Cold brew coffee

Banana

Flax seeds

Cacao nibs

Strawberries

Agave nectar

Cacao powder

AVOCADO TOAST

Whole avocado

Black salt

Bee pollen

Chipotle flakes

ALMOND BUTTER TOAST

Almond butter

Bee pollen

Blueberries

Local honey

PEANUT BUTTER TOAST

Peanut butter

Flax seed

Banana

Local honey

OVERNIGHT OATS

Organic oats

Chia seed

Coconut milk

Honey

Blueberries

Almonds

Granola

Almond butter

More on these and other recipies can be found at
WWW.MYVITALITYPRO.COM or
WWW.FINNSISLANDSTYLEGRUB.COM

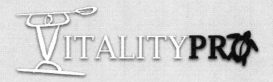

even gain muscle, the calorie total of these two meal installments will be 125 to 150 percent of your usual lunch, with the exercise and fast creating a demand that you're now meeting with a staggered, perfectly timed supply.

Contrast that to overloading your stomach, which has contracted a little during your fast, with a monster shake that's not going to give you the protein-related repair benefits and lacks the types of fats and carbohydrates essential to recovery. Then when you get to your post-fast dinner a few hours later, you're going to want to increase your calories to 125 percent of your typical intake and maintain this throughout the week.

You might be skeptical that you can maintain body weight or even add muscle when you're fasting. This was one of Phil's uncertainties when he first started doing *The 17 Hour Fast*, as he's a lean "hard gainer" who can't afford to lose any muscle. Brandon had similar concerns, though at a jacked 240 pounds, the former lineman has more lean mass than most people. His body weight and composition numbers after fasting weekly for a few months? 235 pounds and a reduction in body fat from 14 percent to 10. So he has actually *increased* his muscle mass while fasting (and he was not even trying to gain muscle during this time). Phil has also put on a few pounds of "good" weight and increased his lean mass. And we've seen this pattern repeated among the Division 1 college athletes and pros who've embraced *The 17 Hour Fast* as part of our VitalityPro camps.

A study conducted by Intermountain Medical Center Heart Institute showed that fasting for 24 hours increases growth hormone in men by up to 2,000 percent and women by 1,300 percent.[58] With our fasting protocol, we hope you're already getting 70.8 percent of that benefit, which is amplified by the way we structure your pre- and post-fast meals. More growth hormone means greater muscle repair and new growth if you're dosing the stimulus and your recovery from it appropriately.

You might notice some early weight loss in the first few weeks as your body sheds some excess body fat. Indeed, research published in *Nature Communications* shows that exercising while fasting helps you burn the dangerous kind of visceral fat that can accumulate around your organs and contribute to metabolic diseases.[59] Another study, conducted by Belgian scientists, found that exercising before breakfast enabled study participants to buffer the effects of overindulging later in the day. Study author Peter Hespel told the *New York Times*, "Only the fasted group demonstrated beneficial metabolic adaptations, which eventually may enhance oxidative fatty acid turnover."[60]

As you're increasing your body's craving for good, clean, whole foods with both exercise and fasting and then meeting these needs on the back end, you will start to reach your body weight, body fat, and muscle mass goals while fasting. And remember that though these can be motivational, the key indicator is how you perform, recover, and feel. Consider writing out your current nutritional approach and jotting a few lines about how you feel during and after workouts, practices, races, or games. Then compare and contrast this to how you feel on fasting days. Yes, you might need to overcome a little wooziness or feeling slightly sluggish the first or second time you fast, but by weeks three and four, your body will be used to running on more ketones and you'll see positive changes in how you perform and feel.

Eliminate Runner's Stomach

For the longest time, people thought that so-called runner's stomach—the bloating, gas bubbles, diarrhea, cramping, and other gastrointestinal symptoms some people experience while completing long-distance runs, rides, or other kinds of endurance work—was brought on by the rigors of the activity itself. This simply isn't true. Most of these complaints are caused by the body trying to pull double duty and focus both on digestion and keeping the body moving. A human body is an amazing thing that's capable of doing many things well, but this kind of super-physiological multitasking isn't on the list.

Earlier, we mentioned the blood flow diversion that occurs when we ingest nutrients while we're training or competing. Though water and electrolytes are necessary for proper hydration and replacement, caloric nutrients introduced into the digestive tract cause a diversion of blood flow away from muscles and vital organs, therefore diminishing performance. Simultaneously, the blood requirement of the muscle and vital organs prevents appropriate blood perfusion of the digestive system to support proper digestion. Therefore, athletic performance and digestion are both compromised.

Many of the gastrointestinal symptoms are related to this hypoperfusion of the digestive tract—a lack of adequate blood flow. Compromised digestion leads to undigested particles of food that act as sponges, retaining water later in the colon. This causes cramping, bloating, and diarrhea. And since the water retained by the undigested food is not properly absorbed by the colon (where the vast majority of water absorption takes place), dehydration sets in.

Training during a fast is one quick and easy way to eliminate the effects of runner's stomach and elevate athletic performance. Exercising while fasting enables your body to focus on the systems that you need to prioritize to go harder, faster, stronger, and longer. We wouldn't suggest that anyone goes to the NFL Combine, the New York Marathon, or an Olympic qualifying event during their first fast, but if you've gotten accustomed to training while fasting over several weeks or months and have maybe tried not eating during a few minor events, you might consider extending the fast to your high-stakes competition. In other words, taper up your training gradually while transitioning into competition.

CAVEAT: Some endurance athletic events such as triathlons, ultra-marathons, etc. will require nutrition during the course of the event. It is the responsibility of the athlete to weigh the cost/benefit ratio, experiment during training, and determine the hydration/nutrition plan that will lead them to success.

LEARNING FROM THE CHAMP: We have learned much from collaborating with many talented athletes. While working as a doctor for the Pipeline Masters surfing championship, Kelly Slater, 11-time world surfing champion, shared with me some of his concepts for hydration/nutrition that sustain him during a full day of competition. One such concept is his use of good fat. He uses avocados as a source of slow and long-burning energy, along with other forms of protein and glucose, which help prevent a fuel crash. A true champion, he continually tweaks and perfects his "recipe."

Pursuing a Tapered Approach

It might be possible for you to jump right into your usual workout during your first fast, and we're not going to tell you that you can't. But a more prudent approach might be to do what you're doing in other phases of the fast and make slow, consistent changes. Remember that fasting itself is a change that your body is confronting, and it's going to take time to get used to fueling activity when you're not eating. Start with a nice long warm-up and then simply do some body weight work like lunges, air squats, push-ups, and so on. Or if you're an endurance athlete, go for a 20- to 30-minute ride, swim, run, or paddle and do it with the same kind of low intensity you do on your "easy" or active recovery days.

Next time you do the fast, crank up the speed, weight, or distance a little bit and see how you feel. Then progress from there, making a conscious effort to be self-aware, and back off a little if you start getting lightheaded or experience any other adverse effects. This gradual, patient approach will enable your muscle cells to take their time in adjusting to the new ketone/glucose mixture you're providing them with and to slowly ramp up as you become more efficient at the cellular level and more confident in your approach. If you follow some of the pointers in the next chapter, you'll also be making improvements to your pre- and post-fast meals, Vacation Night, and Spa Morning that will be beneficial in working out in a semi-ketotic state as well.

When our head trainer, Brandon Rager, was competing in high school, at the Division 1 college level at San Diego State, and in the NFL for the Baltimore Ravens, he tried to boost his output on the game and practice fields and improve his recovery by taking a variety of supplements. "Whey protein and creatine were my go-tos, and everyone else on the team was using them," he said.[61]

Brandon will be one of the first to admit that he was highly skeptical about *The 17 Hour Fast*. He was so used to having some kind of food in his system and then fueling his workouts with supplements that he questioned whether he'd be able to perform in the same way without them. But once he'd tried the fast a few times, he was amazed at the results:

> "I had plenty of energy to get through some hard sessions at the beach and in the pool, and there weren't these big ups and downs like I used to get when I was still playing. There's a level of consistency now that's reassuring because I know that when I'm fasting I'm going to feel great during our VitalityPro camps and am going to be able to coach and train at my best every time."[62]

PART II: MIND AND SOUL

Cognitive Advantage

We've used a lot of ink to share the physical benefits of fasting with you. But athletes and other high performers don't have bodies that function independently. Our every move, thought, and action is controlled by our brain, and fasting can help improve how it functions, adapts, and even grows. We spend much time building our bodies, yet the mind is relatively uncharted territory, which means that improving cognitive performance holds a lot of potential and can become our secret weapon.

In a 2015 TED Talk, Mark Mattson, Chief of the Laboratory of Neurosciences at the National Institute on Aging, told his audience:

> "Challenges to your brain, whether it's intermittent fasting [or] vigorous exercise...are cognitive challenges. When this happens, neuro-circuits are activated, levels of neurotrophic factors increase. That promotes the growth of neurons [and] the formation and strengthening of synapses."[63]

This means that fasting—and, to an even greater degree, exercising while fasting—can stimulate brain development and improve the speed at which messages are transmitted within and across certain brain regions. No wonder that I feel like I'm a better doctor while I'm fasting. In an interview for the Florida Institute for Human and Machine Cognition's STEM-Talk podcast, Mattson went on to say that fasting boosts the release of beta-hydroxybutyrate, which stimulates production of brain-derived neurotrophic factor. This plays a key role in memory, learning new skills, and improving existing ones.[64] It is also involved in growing new cells (aka neurogenesis) in the hippocampus, one of the brain regions responsible for governing mood and spatial navigation.

Speaking of the hippocampus, another neurologist, Dr. Sandrine Thuret from King's College, agrees with Mattson that fasting can help generate new cells in this region of the brain. This is supported by the work of neuroscientist Eleanor Maguire of University College London, who found that London taxi drivers have a larger hippocampus than most people, likely because their brain has to grow to remember and quickly recall the possible routes through the bustling city's 25,000 streets.[65]

Thuret states that learning and exercise can play a role in increasing neurogenesis in this region of the brain, as can fasting. "Calorie restriction of 20 to 30 percent will increase neurogenesis, and so will fasting...spacing the time between your meals," she said in a presentation in London.[66] So in this way, limiting your calorie intake with the fast itself and also reducing calorie intake in your pre- and post-fast meals may actually make your brain grow in ways that will improve how you move through the world spatially and emotionally. Even if you're not going to be driving a taxi, Thuret suggests that such brain cell growth could help with everyday tasks like finding your bike that you've left in a crowded train station. Or, in Phil's case, giving him back all that time he wastes each week searching frantically for his keys and wallet.

Fasting also provides some much-needed housekeeping inside your head. We mentioned earlier how doing *The 17 Hour Fast* encourages your body to flush out the overgrowth of bad bacteria and kill off dead or dying cells.[67] One study published in *Autophagy* found that this is also the case with brain cells. A group of Chinese researchers discovered that fasting reduces oxidative stress that can damage neural cells (which might be what's going on when we get so-called brain fog) and, if left unchecked, eventually may contribute to cognitive decline.[68]

No matter what your field is, it's becoming increasingly clear that fasting gives your brain a workout that prompts it to become more elastic, higher functioning, better able to grow and regenerate, and more resistant to cellular damage. That's going to give you an edge on the football field, in the classroom, and in the boardroom, both now and over the long term. And the best thing about this? Because these benefits aren't physically apparent, your competitors will never see you coming.

Boost Your Brainpower

We've talked a lot about how having slightly more ketones can help you improve your physical performance. But that isn't the only way that *The 17 Hour Fast* can give you a natural advantage. When we're learning new skills and honing existing ones, our body uses a fatty substance called myelin to improve the speed at which certain regions of our brain communicate and access these skills.

Myelin is made of fat, so you need fat to build and reinforce it. Some of us get insufficient ketone bodies to power this process, and if the brain recognizes that it's running low on fuel, it can start gobbling up myelin to supply more energy. By switching the macronutrient composition of your pre- and post-fast lunches and dinners and replacing some sugar calories with those derived from fats and leucine and lysine amino acids, you're giving your brain better building blocks to make myelin and so support brain-based skill adaptations.[69]

A study published in *Neurobiology of Aging* reveals that increasing ketone levels helps people with Alzheimer's and other cognitive conditions improve their memory, suggesting that it can provide similar benefits to those who don't have such a disease.[70] Dr. William Lagakos, an expert in inflammation and insulin resistance and author of *The Poor, Misunderstood Calorie* also believes that giving the brain more ketones can help alleviate so-called brain fog by improving the regulation of GABA and glutamate.[71] So if you start creating more ketones through fasting and changing the composition of your meals, you're going to be getting a brain boost as well as a physical one.

The Gift of Calm and Clarity

One of the elite performers who has found great success with fasting at least once a week is a high-powered business executive I know. Everyone who meets him is impressed by his confidence and the sense of command he seems to have over any given situation. But little do many people know that he's terrified of public speaking. One time his company scheduled him to be the main speaker at its board meeting. He emailed me to say that he had been planning to fast that day but wasn't sure he should because he was worried it might make him feel more nervous. I assured him that fasting actually makes me steadier when I'm going into a shift in the ER.

So he went ahead and did *The 17 Hour Fast*. I emailed him to see how his talk went and how he felt before and during his presentation (with fingers crossed that everything had gone well). He told me that he was amazed by the sense of tranquility he felt in the few minutes leading up to it, and that he had an unusually high level of focus as he was working through his

PowerPoint deck. So now anytime he has to meet with the board, investors, or big clients, he's doing *The 17 Hour Fast.* We've heard many similar stories from the EMTs, firefighters, and police officers who've attended VitalityPro camps and started doing the fast. Lives are on the line each and every time they report for duty, and they tell me that they feel calmer and better able to manage their adrenaline when they're fasting.

One time when I was volunteering as a doctor on site at a Triple Crown surfing event, one of the competitors tried to grab a jersey away from another surfer. Other people got involved, and it quickly escalated. I vividly remember how Randy Rarick, who was director of the Triple Crown at the time, handled the situation. A lot of people would have charged in and started shouting or even pushing and shoving. Not Randy. He calmly took the jersey from the guy who was all fired up and ready to fight and gave it back to the other surfer. This display of calm under pressure completely defused this heated situation without the need for any physicality or harsh words.

I visualize this scene sometimes when it gets hectic in the emergency room. Rather than yelling and rushing around, I've found that it makes me more efficient and calms the others down if I talk a little quieter, slower, and try to be more methodical in setting a tone of calm rather than one of panic. Here's Randy's take:

"It gives people strength when you can show them that someone's in control of a situation. One time I was running a tournament at Waimea and this Brazilian surfer got pounded by a 25-foot set. Everyone went nuts. People were coming up to me screaming, 'You've got to stop this thing. Someone's gonna get killed out there.' I just told them very calmly that the lifeguards were taking care of the guy and that we were going to wait for a few minutes and see what happened with the conditions. While everyone else was speeding up, I slowed down and this rubbed off on my staff and the spectators. When things get chaotic, you need to project order and that you're in command, even if you have to fake it a little bit sometimes."[72]

Upgrade Your Life

The bigger the stressor you're exposed to, the greater your need for recovery. And the more frequently you're exposed to high demands on your body and mind, the more often you need premium rest. The trouble is that although high performers are typically proficient at revving up to face the rigors that each day brings, they're sometimes guilty of not allowing themselves appropriate downtime to revitalize.

This is why *The 17 Hour Fast* is so useful for those who regularly push the limits. It can provide the chance to reset and reboot, not just because of the myriad benefits that fasting offers but also due to the habits it encourages you to create during those 17 hours. First off, the Vacation Night is the perfect chance to reconnect with friends who are usually left by the wayside as you're off pursuing your goals. It's also the chance to make time for your family members, who might often feel like they've been relegated down the priorities pecking order. Then when you get to the Spa Morning, if you're able to resist the temptation of plugging back in and resuming your usual hectic pace, you'll find that you can start making more space for yourself. This involves adding in time for reflection and thinking ahead that you probably rarely get, reconnecting with the natural world, and either starting a discipline like meditation, prayer, or journaling for the first time or picking it back up again after a potentially long hiatus. To stay at the top, you're going to have to start building things like this into your daily routine and not just on the days that you're fasting. And there's no better time than now to begin.

Winning with Intangibles

Going into halftime of Super Bowl 51, the New England Patriots trailed the Atlanta Falcons by the seemingly insurmountable margin of 21-3. The underdogs from the South had surprised Bill Belichick's squad by coming out with intensity and determination that perhaps they didn't expect, and it showed on the scoreboard. Almost everyone watching had written the Pats off by this point. Surely this team and its 40-year-old quarterback didn't have the energy to come back from such a deficit, not with the Falcons riding the confidence wave of their offensive barrage and a series of crushing defensive stops.

The second half didn't go any better for New England, which soon found itself in a 25-point hole, down 28-3. But just as it seemed that Brady and his squad were done for, they flipped the script and mounted one of the most spirited comebacks in the history of the sport. One incredible offensive drive after another saw the Patriots score 31 unanswered points, with their seemingly indefatigable quarterback leading the charge to the unlikeliest of wins in overtime. By now, most people know Brady's story. Despite having a solid college career at the University of Michigan, his NFL Combine performance was underwhelming and he slipped to the very last pick of the draft.

Undeterred, Coach Belichick selected Brady and was quickly impressed by how hard the young man, who was supposedly too weak, too small, and too slow to succeed in the pro game, worked, how late he stayed most nights to throw extra passes, and how diligently he studied film and the playbook. When the team lost starting quarterback Drew Bledsoe in the second game of the 2001 season, Brady seized his chance and the starter's job, and then went on to win two league MVPs, four Super Bowl MVPs, and five championships, including that remarkable back-from-the-dead performance in Super Bowl 51.

One of the things that scouts didn't see in Brady isn't measurable in the weight room, in the 40-yard dash, or in the vertical leap test: "intangibles." In the case of the almost undrafted quarterback, these included a dedication to maintaining his overall health, an underrated tactical acumen, and as we know, an unbreakable will. Yes, there are some high performers who get by on physical or mental gifts, pure talent, or privilege. But there are just as many whose ability to do the little things well sets them apart, even when nobody initially recognizes their potential for greatness.

We're not guaranteeing that *The 17 Hour Fast* will take a bench warmer and make them an All Star, will help a business owner turn a struggling company into a Fortune 500 giant, or will enable a starving artist to become the next Picasso. But it will give you an unseen performance advantage in the "intangibles" by providing your body and brain with a long-lasting blend of ketones and glucose, calming down your nervous system, and enabling you to transfer the discipline and self-control it takes to fast to what you do best.

Hard-Driving = Hard-Crashing

If you drive a car at 30 miles an hour and hit something, it's going to be a problem. Going 90? You're probably not walking away. The motivation and relentless ambition that fuels high performers to excel can also be their greatest weakness, as they don't know when or how to take their foot off the gas pedal. Often it takes an acute event like a heart attack, a chronic issue like adrenal fatigue, or a break in a relationship to force such hard drivers to slow down.

Then we add in devices that make us always available to colleagues, put our email a single click away, and allow us to use productivity apps from any device, anywhere, at any time. This means that we might physically leave the office, the military base, or the lecture hall behind at the end of the day, but our work follows us home and wherever else we go. As a result, many of us never truly unwind because we're never fully disconnected from our responsibilities. And as we all have endless to-do lists, there's always something we could (and often feel we should) be doing.

I remember that when I started practicing medicine, I used to have a pager that the hospital could use to reach me if they needed me to come in and cover a colleague's shift. Other than me and my fellow doctors, the only people I knew who could be summoned in this way were police officers and firefighters. Now that cell phones are so pervasive (not to mention call- and text-enabled watches, fitness trackers, and other devices), we're all contactable at all times. So when we're trying to help a high performer get the most out of *The 17 Hour Fast,* one of the first things we advise them to do is to strategically turn off their phone at certain times of day and, when possible, during the Vacation Night and Spa Morning.

Whatever that email, text, or voicemail is about can usually wait until the next day. If you're someone who honestly says they need to be more in touch than that, then resolve to turn your device back on for just a couple of minutes per hour or every few hours. But don't do so unless you absolutely have to, and have the self-control to immediately hit the off button afterward. Yes, we did introduce this concept of a tech fast in the Vacation Night chapter, but for business executives, creatives, and other high performers, tech addiction and being tethered to obligations is an even greater challenge, so it bears repeating.

Our good friend Peter Furler travels a lot in his dual role of musician and producer. When we asked him about his routine the day after coming back from a road trip, he told us, "I switch off my phone and don't even open my laptop. I need that whole day to devote to my family. When I was younger,

I used to think that to be productive I had to be connected 24/7. Now I've learned that you can never finish every task and that work can wait. I'm doing less now and think that my work is higher quality than ever."[73]

Attitude is Everything

We've already mentioned the confidence Brandon gets to train clients while he's fasting, the even keel I'm on while doing *The 17 Hour Fast* in the emergency room, and the calm my CEO friend experiences with the fast. Phil achieves the same laser-like focus when he's writing. All of us have seen the benefits of fasting firsthand. Maybe you still have some anxieties because you've only done the fast once or haven't tried it yet. If that's the case, go into your workout, meeting, test, or whatever during your fast with a positive, can-do attitude. If you tell yourself, "I'm going to feel great and ace this," and your posture, words, and actions mirror such a mindset, you will most likely be successful. In contrast, if you go in with fear and trembling or thinking skeptically that there's no way you can perform while fasting, guess what? You'll probably have a bad experience.

By choosing thoughtfully how to set your attitude, your demeanor, and your expectations, you'll go a long way in determining the results of your fast and whatever situations you find yourself in during it. A good friend once told me, "Whether you think you'll win or lose, you'll be right." Or in other words, to a large extent, we live out our "self-fulfilling prophecies." Positivity, optimism, and confidence are contagious. Combine these with the ketone clarity we mentioned earlier and you have a pretty potent blueprint to get ahead, no matter what your game, job, degree, or vocation is.

Challenge Yourself

One of the best things about hard-charging people is that they're always up for a new challenge, whether that's in their career, their hobbies, or any other part of their life. High achievers are never satisfied with the status quo and are constantly looking for ways to stretch themselves. Sound familiar? Good! Then I want you to look at *The 17 Hour Fast* as a challenge that you will need commitment, determination, and stick-to-it-iveness to attempt and then, once you've done it the first time, to perfect (see the next chapter).

In a Facebook post about fasting, CrossFit mindset coach and founder of The Alpha Movement Tom Foxley wrote:

> "Perseverance, determination, and grit are transferable skills. On top of this, there's nothing innate about them. You can learn them through practicing. We should go out of our way to eradicate sustained comfort. Or at least put ourselves through temporary levels of intense discomfort. As with most of these temporary discomforts, the result is a positive one—both mentally and physically. About 14 hours into this fast, I was already irritable, craving any food and losing focus easily. Pushing through this phase was tough. But here's the thing: by practicing this fortitude, we build a baseline of resilience."[74]

In addition to practicing perseverance through your fast, you can also embrace the leadership challenge it presents. If you're married, you can lead the way for your spouse. You can also be a positive influence on your parents, siblings, cousins, other family members, and friends, some of whom might be in desperate need of the positive lifestyle changes that *The 17 Hour Fast* can deliver. If you're used to leading a group of soldiers, a company, a sports team, or any other group, put those leadership and motivational qualities to good use here as well.

Creating a 26-and-1/4-Hour Day

What's the deal with this subhead? It seems a little silly, we'll admit. No, we're not claiming that we can actually bend the space-time continuum with *The 17 Hour Fast*. But there are ways that it gives you more of our greatest commodity. In our research, we've found that the typical person who follows our protocol gains back around 2.25 hours when they do the fast, by not shopping for, preparing, eating, clearing up, or thinking about food. Peter Furler told us about how he reallocates such time:

> "Instead of hunting out more food at the supermarket, I track down a good book instead. Then I sit down with it, get a pencil to make notes, and start working through it. I look at reading as a treat for myself. It's a way to gain knowledge and also to wind down. If you look at the habits of high achievers, most of them get up early, are active, and read every day."[75]

Additionally, we can add days to our lives. Truthfully, each decision we make, such as jogging a mile or eating that candy bar, adds to or subtracts from our health and life span. So appropriate interval fasting can add health and therefore days to your life.

A New Kind of Leadership

If you're an executive, a pro athlete, a police chief, a military officer, or another authority figure, you're used to being in charge most of the time. And yet in my experience, such people can have trouble with the group-oriented aspects of *The 17 Hour Fast* initially. Whether it's carving out time to spend on a family game night or going out with friends for a distraction-free dinner, high achievers often find it difficult to fully disconnect from their day-to-day responsibilities and fully engage with the people they care about.

If that sounds all too familiar, do something you probably rarely do: ask for help. It's not a sign of shortcoming or weakness, but rather a sign of self-awareness. If I've had an intense shift in the ER, my thoughts are sometimes still circling the ceiling when I begin my fast. So I ask Regina to take the lead and plan something that will help me relax, put my hard day in the rearview mirror, and fully switch my focus back to her and our kids. If you ask for help, your spouse, fiancé, friend, or whoever you choose to team up with will almost certainly be willing to initiate your Vacation Night, taking yet another burden off you and helping you ease into a much-needed night of restoration.

The Highest of High Performers

We've already shared some insights from Coach Gene Stallings and how his winning mindset transcended the football field. Another important lesson we can learn from the Stallings family comes from his son John Mark, who was born with Down syndrome. In his wonderful book *Another Season,* Coach Stallings reveals that at the time, some people chose not to keep children with this condition. He and his wife, Ruth Ann, not only kept John Mark but became pioneers by bringing their beloved son into the "mainstream." This led to the expansion of the RISE program, which the Stallings family helped grow from a tiny, one-room operation into a state-of-the-art center on the University of Alabama campus and six other integrative schools where children with Down syndrome and other special needs learn alongside their peers who don't have such conditions.

John Mark didn't just influence the expansion of the RISE program but also the lives of the football team, Alabama fans, and the thousands of visitors he guided through the Paul "Bear" Bryant Museum, named in honor of Coach Stallings's legendary first boss. "Johnny loved to go to work every day, was never late, and rarely called in sick," Coach Stallings said. "He really earned that paycheck. Many people asked him to lead them around the Bryant Museum, and when he was done, he'd come take a nap on the couch in my office. Then we'd go out to practice together."[76] John Mark positively impacted everyone he met, his father revealed: "It didn't matter if you were the richest person or the poorest person, you were important to him and you were his friend. His love was unconditional."[77]

The way John Mark cared for and inspired others is memorialized in Faulkner University's stadium, which was unveiled as John Mark Stallings Field in 2010. He also has a street named after him on the University of Alabama campus, as well as the playground behind the RISE Center that he and his family raised funds for. To us, he is the ultimate high performer.

John Mark's legacy has also had a profound personal impact on me. Earlier this year, I received a call from Bay High School. They had a team of children eagerly looking forward to competing in the Special Olympics but couldn't find a doctor in time to perform the required health screenings. I was very busy with my work at the hospital and VitalityPro but immediately agreed to help. It soon became clear that these screenings were going to take a "little" longer than usual because as I tried to check many of the children's ears or eyes, they repeatedly threw their arms around me in a strong hug. I thought, "This may take a while, but slow down and enjoy these kids." So rather than feeling rushed, I relished these displays of affection. When I'd finished all the screenings and cleared the kids to participate, they were overjoyed that they were going to be able to compete that Friday. It was a joy to watch people clapping and cheering for them from the stands. I'm grateful for the opportunity to work with elite athletes, but my two most cherished sporting experiences in the past year have been coaching my sons' soccer team and helping those kids realize their Special Olympics dreams.

PERFECTING YOUR FAST

The first time someone runs a marathon, they just want to finish. Sure, they might have a generic time goal, but for the most part, just getting across the line is satisfaction enough. You should have the same mindset with your initial fast. First of all, be proud of yourself for getting this far and having the willpower to see it through.

Now it's time to get even better. After a marathon runner has finished the 26.2 mile course, they sit with their coach and break down the race. What went right and what went wrong? Did they nail the hydration plan or finish the course feeling like a dried-out husk? Was their nutrition strategy on point or did it leave them feeling ragged for those last few agonizing miles? Did they choose the right shoes, or did a seam rub their toes raw? And so on.

We want you to do the same post-event analysis after completing your first *17 Hour Fast*. You likely nailed a few elements, so well done. But what didn't go so well? Maybe your sleep hygiene wasn't great so you felt too wired to fall asleep. Perhaps you didn't drink enough water. You might have made the mistake of stressing yourself out with a work project or by watching news footage of a natural disaster.

This is one of the areas in which *The 17 Hour Fast* is very different from other fasting programs. They typically require you to add more, usually by increasing the number of hours that you go without food. But as Steve Jobs rightly said, "Simple can be harder than complex: You have to work hard to get your thinking clean to make it simple."[78] We've spent years working with our multidisciplinary team at VitalityPro to clean up our thinking on fasting and put all of our research into the simplest system possible, which makes it easier for you to achieve even greater success with your second, third, and fourth fasts. And the good news is that we're not asking you to add more hours—in fact, not even an extra minute. Instead, see what you can remove or tweak to enhance your experience and increase the benefits you get.

Of course, to improve on your first attempt and begin refining your approach, you're going to have to take another crack at it. And as anyone who has learned an instrument, trained for a sport, or dedicated themselves to a creative pursuit like painting or writing knows, consistency is key. So the next step is to commit to doing *The 17 Hour Fast* weekly. Eventually you might find you want to do it more often, as we do. But like we just wrote, this is not a book about doing things more but about doing them better. So for now, just try for once a week. Once you've resolved to do the fast weekly, an easy way to start your post-fast review is to work through it chronologically, just as we've structured this book. So let's break down what happened:

A. Pre-Fast Meals

Did you set yourself up for success with your routines before the fast began? In your pre-fast lunch and dinner, did you manage to get your carbs down to 30 and 20 percent, respectively? If so, that's excellent. Now let's make sure that this percentage is comprised of good, low-glycemic foods like vegetables, low-sugar fruits, and whole grains like oats, quinoa, and brown rice. If not, don't worry. Let's take your actual pre-fast meal carb count and cut it by 5 to 10 percent next time. If you gorged yourself because you were worried you wouldn't have sufficient fuel to make it to the finish, remember that your liver can produce enough ketones and glucose to keep you alive and thriving for days on end. It's also important to go into your fast well hydrated, so bear that in mind for next time if you ended up feeling parched at any point.

Outside of pre-fast meal nutrition and hydration, try to pinpoint anything else in the hours that preceded the fast that might have sabotaged you. If you got less than six hours of sleep the night before the fasting night, then you were already more insulin resistant than normal and also were less effi-cient and effective at metabolizing fat. Resolve to get a longer, higher qual-ity night's rest before you start your second fast.

B. Vacation Night

Were you all in when creating a stress-free experience for yourself and your family, or did you just stick to your normal routine? If it was the latter, try to list the stressors you felt and set up conditions to eliminate them next time. How was your hydration that night? If you drank enough water, good for you. If not, try to add in another glass next time. Did you drink too much water and wake up to go to the restroom too much? Did you make an effort to taper down your sleep aid, caffeine, and alcohol? Two thumbs up if you were able to do so. Aim to cut back a little more next time. If you did-n't, we're not judging you. Just try to reduce your intake for your second fast. Remember that we're still trying to improve our own fasting routines and will never be done tweaking the recipe. Apply the same continual growth mindset to your own self-experimentation.

C. Ketotic Sleep

How did you sleep during the initial fast? Perhaps you stayed asleep all night and woke up feeling about the same or even better than normal. Nicely done! But if you had frequent interruptions and got out of bed wishing you could have another couple of hours of shut eye, you probably need to change something. Was your room cold enough, did you avoid blue and harsh LED lights before bedtime, and did you relax with a massage, breathing work, and/or mobility exercises? Consider adding in these game changers if you didn't already try them.

Also think about whether you started your fast at the right time to suit your lifestyle and chronotype (i.e., whether you're naturally predisposed to being a night owl or an early bird). As we wrote earlier, your physiology is not the same as mine or Phil's and beginning *The 17 Hour Fast* at 7 PM and end-ing it at noon the next day is just a suggestion. If you're a night owl like Phil who's usually up until midnight or later, then the chances are that starting the fast at 7 PM and trying to go to sleep at 9 or 10 PM didn't work for you because the change from your normal routine was too great. Similarly, if you're a super early bird like me, you might need to start your fast before that suggested 7 PM kickoff time and go to bed earlier to account for your early rising habit. There is no "good" or "bad" here—just tinker with the timing and figure out what helps you achieve reparative and uninterrupted sleep.

D. Spa Morning

When you were in the last stage of your fast, did you maintain your feeling of calm and relaxation from the Vacation Night? If not, what happened to disrupt it? Of course, there are unexpected life events—getting called into work because a colleague is out sick, receiving bad news about a family member, and so on—that we can't anticipate. But outside of these random occurrences, did you do everything you could to control the more predictable elements of your morning and create conditions for a pleasant experience?

If not, what could you have done differently? Sometimes it's as easy as doing a few minutes of extra planning during your Vacation Night so you're scheduling Spa Morning activities you enjoy and avoiding situations that can irritate, frustrate, or upset you. If events seem to conspire against you, recognize that while you might not be able to eliminate random occurrences, you *can* control how you react to them. Instead of letting your initial reaction of shock, panic, or despondency take hold, try to delay responding until you've got your emotions and attitude in check. If you can smile at the absurdity of the situation and take a few deep breaths, you can still come away with a positive experience.

We often feel pressured to give people who come to our VitalityPro camps a perfect day, which many times coincides with our own mid-fast Spa Morning. Yet sometimes the elements don't cooperate and we have an unusually cold day or heavy rain that forces us to change the program. If we start sweating about what these college coaches, big-time business executives, and our other clients will think of us, we can begin to panic. But we have to remember that we can be a thermostat—something that senses the environment and adjusts the conditions to make them more pleasant— rather than a thermometer, which only reacts to the given environment. Be a thermostat!

If you worked during your Spa Morning, try to see if you made use of the ketone clarity that fasting can provide. For most of the high performers we collaborate with, this means blocking off an hour to 90 minutes for focused attention on a single project. Did you do that or spend most of your time clearing out your inbox or, dare we say, browsing the web? If it's the latter, make a real effort to be more self-controlled and intentional next time.

E. Post-Fast Meals

When you looked at the clock and saw that your first *17 Hour Fast* was over, did you allow yourself to celebrate? Some of us, particularly hard-driving, type-A personalities, find it hard to let ourselves do this as we're looking ahead to the next thing. If this is you, make an effort to be fully present next time and give yourself a well-deserved pat on the back. The next consideration is your post-fast lunch and dinner. Did you keep your portion size small and focus mainly on high quality fats, lean proteins, and vegetables? If so, keep doing what you're doing. If you got a giant meal at a fast food drive-through to celebrate, consider going with a healthier option and smaller quantity after your second fast.

Also think about the pace of your post-fast meals. Did you savor each bite as you enjoyed the company of family and friends or grab takeout that you hurriedly ate at your desk while catching up on work tasks? Were you able to create a gap in your schedule to ease into the rest of the day, or did you go right back to rushing around? Try to extend the mood you created during your Vacation Night and carried into the Spa Morning for as long as possible and, like Randy Rarick, avoid hurrying when possible to keep stress and anxiety at bay.

LIMIT THE VARIABLES

One of the biggest mistakes we can make when tweaking and improving our fasting and the habits, rituals, and practices that surround it is to give into the temptation of overcomplication. Because we've been conditioned to always go further, faster, and heavier in the gym, to squeeze every last drop of productivity out of ourselves at work and in school, and to load up our social calendars to the max, the natural tendency is to apply this line of thinking to the fast. But if you do, you're not going to get the across-the-board results you want. When people first come to us at VitalityPro, the athletes and high performers we talked about in the previous chapter typically want to improve everything in their workouts and their business and private lives. As a result, they prioritize nothing and make very minimal improvements in each of their target areas.

Any performance specialist or coach worth their salt will tell you that you shouldn't try to boost speed, power, endurance, and every other physical quality in all your workouts. It will either overload you, meaning that you underdevelop each of these characteristics, or make it very difficult to recover adequately. Great coaches attempt to address one or two variables at the most each training session. The same is true in your office or classroom. If you go in and try to optimize every single thing all at once, your scattershot approach will make you lose sight of your primary objectives and make it hard to achieve specific goals. And even if you do see an overall improvement, because you're changing so many variables, it will be nearly impossible to know which one led to the positive change. Or on the flipside, if all you get is a net negative, you'll struggle to see which alteration is at the root of the issue.

A more effective and manageable way ahead is to simply identify one thing you want to improve in each area that we've touched upon in this book. And make sure that the changes you're making are incremental and realistically achievable. So if you're used to eating lunches and dinners comprised of 80 percent carbs, don't immediately shoot for cutting this down to 30 percent. Otherwise you're going to create a stressor because the differential between where you were and where you are now is too great. So in this case, aim for dialing back the carbs to 70 percent in your first crack at *The 17 Hour Fast,* then 60 in the second attempt, and 50 in the third. You're on the right track.

You might not always see a linear progression because that's not how life or your body works. So you may be fine at that 50 percent carb level but have a bad experience when you dial back the percentage again to 40. In which case, try going to 45 percent the next time you fast. Still feel lousy? Then stick with 50 and change another variable instead. Only you are you, so there cannot be a broad-strokes approach that is inflexible and infallible for all people.

In keeping with the action plan we suggested writing down during your Spa Morning, be intentional here and write out your goals for your second fast in a notebook or on your phone, tablet, or computer. You can then scribble some brief thoughts on what went well, what didn't, and whether you're going to keep tweaking this variable in weeks three, four, and five or switch to another. Here's an example of how your plan for your second fast might look:

PRE-FAST MEALS

Variable: Macronutrient breakdown

Week 2 goal: Reduce carbs to 40 percent

Week 2 post-fast notes: Felt great! Try to cut pre-fast meal carbs to 30 percent next week.

VACATION NIGHT

Variable: Time with friends or family

Week 2 goal: Add another 15 minutes of protected time

Week 2 post-fast notes: Didn't go well because I forgot to turn my phone off. Try again next week.

KETOTIC SLEEP

Variable: Bedtime

Week 2 goal: Go to bed 15 minutes earlier

Week 2 post-fast notes: Adjustment went smoothly. Shoot for going to bed another 15 minutes earlier next time.

SPA MORNING

Variable: Volunteering

Week 2 goal: Increase time at homeless shelter from 30 minutes to an hour

Week 2 post-fast notes: Rewarding time at the shelter today! Sign up again for next week.

POST-FAST MEALS

Variable: Meal composition

Week 2 goal: Add in another vegetable to post-fast lunch

Week 2 post-fast notes: Chopped up some carrots for my salad, and it tasted even better. Try adding another veggie next week.

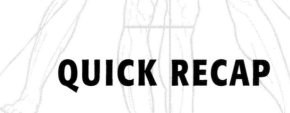

QUICK RECAP

CHAPTER 12

If you read every chapter straight through, most of it might still be fresh in your mind. But it's easy to get waylaid and read a book in chunks over several weeks or have multiple titles on your nightstand at once that you read a little bit from here and there. That's why we want to quickly recap the main stages of *The 17 Hour Fast*. Remember to visit our social media pages to share your experiences, interact with other fasters, and ask questions. Please use the hashtag #17hourfast when you post so we can find your message and, when we're able, respond to you. Thank you again for your willingness to stick with this book and use it to positively change your lifestyle and impact others, both by protecting your time with family and friends and participating in the Calorie and Goodwill Exchange program.

Now on to the quick recap:

1. HEALTH SCREEN AND COLLABORATIVE MODEL

- Schedule an appointment with your primary care physician. If you don't have one, choose a doctor who matches your interests and values.

- Get testing/screening done, including height, weight and body mass index (BMI), body fat percentage, resting blood pressure, resting respiratory rate (oxygen saturation), and resting heart rate. Add in any other tests and screenings your doctor recommends, which may include complete blood count, chemistry panel, thyroid panel, lipid and hormone panels, and possibly colonoscopy, mammogram, or prostate screen.

- Get clearance from your doctor before starting the fast.

- If your doctor doesn't give you the go-ahead to fast initially, you can still benefit from many of the accompanying lifestyle principles.

- Write down your personal and family medical histories, vital sign benchmarks, blood sugar levels, etc. and put this information in your wallet or purse. You could also add this data into the health app or notes section on your phone.

- Once you've done the fast for at least 12 weeks, have a follow-up appointment with your physician for appropriate retesting, and follow their advice regarding any adjustments.

2. PRE-FAST MEALS

PRE-FAST LUNCH

Fat: 35 percent   *Protein:* 35 percent   *Carbs:* 30 percent
Calories: 50 to 75 percent of usual lunch

PRE-FAST DINNER

Fat: 40 percent   *Protein:* 40 percent   *Carbs:* 20 percent
Calories: 50 to 75 percent of usual dinner

3. VACATION NIGHT

- Block off dedicated time to spend with family members and/or friends.

- Try doing a technology fast at the same time to improve your focus, increase self-discipline, and avoid food-based advertising.

- Do some mobility, massage, and/or soft tissue work.

- Don't do any work or look at anything that might cause stress, like the news, stock market report, or bills.

- Go "analog" and play board games, put on some music, or go bowling.
- Try immersing yourself in water to improve relaxation.

4. KETOTIC SLEEP

- Avoid screens that give off blue light before bed.
- Read a book.
- Perform a breathing routine such as the one mentioned earlier to help you relax.
- Improve your existing sleep hygiene routine or create a new one, including sleeping with the thermostat set a little cooler, removing electronic devices from your bedroom, blocking out light and noise, etc.
- Go to bed 30 minutes earlier after planning out your Spa Morning.

5. SPA MORNING

- Get up 30 minutes earlier than usual.
- Take a few minutes to be thankful.
- If you're working, make an effort to block off time for important projects.
- Do some mobility work, and if you can, get a massage or other spa treatment.
- Perform a breathing routine.
- Devote 30 to 60 minutes to self-reflection, meditation, or prayer and develop an action plan that will enable you to meet an ambitious goal.
- Spend some time outdoors in nature.
- If you're an athlete, start with a light workout and gradually progress as your body gets used to your new ketone/glucose flex fuel.
- Help change the lives of those with water- and food-related needs by supporting the Calorie and Goodwill Exchange program at www.17hourfast.com/charities and supporting non-profits like Food for the Hungry, The Last Well, Strikeouts for Troops, World Vision, and others.

6. POST-FAST MEALS

POST-FAST LUNCH

Fat: 40 percent   *Protein:* 40 percent   *Carbs:* 20 percent

Calories: 50 to 75 percent of usual lunch

POST-FAST DINNER

Fat: 35 percent   *Protein:* 35 percent   *Carbs:* 30 percent

Calories: 75 percent of usual dinner. If you're at a healthy BMI/body fat percentage/weight, return to 100 percent of usual meals starting with the next meal, which should be breakfast. If you're trying to lose weight, try to stick with this 75 percent for each subsequent meal for as long as you can.

7. FASTING FOR HIGH PERFORMANCE

- Combine exercise and fasting for a potent, brain- and body-boosting combination.

- Use the fast to achieve ketone clarity for important projects and to remain calm when public speaking or in other stressful situations.

- Help ensure success with a positive mental attitude.

- Recognize that any anxiety you might have about not having adequate fuel for your workout is mostly a psychological barrier, and then change your expectations to positive ones.

- Use the fast as an opportunity to set and reinforce stronger boundaries between your work and family life and to better organize and prioritize your time.

- Look at *The 17 Hour Fast* as a new challenge—and remember to celebrate when you succeed.

- Athletes, use the following post-fast meal breakdown to help maintain or gain muscle:

POST-FAST LUNCH PART ONE

Fat: 40 percent   *Protein:* 40 percent   *Carbs:* 20 percent

Calories: 75 to 100 percent of usual lunch

POST-FAST LUNCH PART TWO/SNACK (approx. two hours after lunch)

Fat: 10 percent   *Protein:* 70 percent   *Carbs:* 20 percent

Calories: 50 percent of usual lunch

(total of 125 to 150 percent when combined with post-fast lunch part one)

POST-FAST DINNER

Fat: 40 percent   *Protein:* 40 percent   *Carbs:* 20 percent

Calories: 100 to 125 percent of usual dinner. Try to keep the 125 percent calories going for as many meals as possible to fuel muscle gain.

8. PERFECTING THE FAST

- Commit to fasting at least once a week, every week.

- Ask a family member or friend to fast with you to improve accountability.

- Pick one variable you can improve for each element of the main *17 Hour Fast* stages each week.

- Instead of creating large or dramatic changes, try to make gradual, sustainable ones.

- Don't try to just add more, but resolve to do certain things better (like protecting family time).

- Remedy any issues you had, like letting work intrude on your Vacation Night.

- If you broke the fast early, try to add a little more time each week until you get to 17 hours.

- Be your own experiment and keep tweaking the fasting recipe to get the best results for you.

- Share what works and what doesn't with us and fellow readers on our our social channels using the hashtag #17hourfast.

FULFILLING THE PROMISE

We started this book with a promise to my friend Jason and in memory of Phil's father-in-law, John. We've poured 15 years of research, hundreds of hours, and dozens of late nights into this book, not to mention more tears than we care to count. It has been a humbling pursuit of a commitment. We hope that *The 17 Hour Fast* improves your health, enhances your quality of life, and empowers you to help others. We hope Jason and John are proud of us.

POSTSCRIPT

NOVEMBER 15, 2017

I started writing this book with Phil from my home in Florida, edited it during a sabbatical in Malibu, California, and now close it from Haiti. I'm writing this while taking malaria prophylactic medicine and under a mosquito net on a medical mission with Live Beyond. Why leave affluent coastal America for one of the most disease- and poverty-stricken areas in the world?

Because I have grown as a person while collectively working on *The 17 Hour Fast* with Phil, our wives, and our friends and contributors. Phil tells me it's changed him too. Most of the individuals we've collaborated with on the book have expressed the same sentiment.

How have we changed? We cherish life more and therefore love more. With deeper love, we take purposeful and directed action to be with and help others, both in our relationships with loved ones and with total strangers in our communities and abroad.

I'll end with this story.

Yesterday, while I was missing my wife and sons, I saw a Haitian boy at our church service wearing an old Alabama jersey (my boys love Alabama football). This young man knew nothing about my home state or my family's favorite college football team, but I recognized that this encounter was more than a coincidence. Later that day, David and Laura Vanderpool, who run Live Beyond, took us to the boy's home where we met his mother and seven siblings. The conditions were below what we'd consider acceptable for humans or animals in the US, like in most of this impoverished nation. My heart stirred with emotion. This was no time for compassion fatigue. It was time for action. After a brief talk with David, my family decided to partner with Live Beyond to fund a new home for them.

You see, *The 17 Hour Fast* isn't just about resetting your relationship to food or carving out more "me time." It's much bigger than that. God used my writing this book, Coach Stallings's encouragement to me to go to Haiti, and an old Alabama jersey to bring aid and hope to the oppressed. May you be similarly blessed as you experience personal growth and take decisive action to improve the lives of others. We can't wait to hear your stories.

Humbly,

FRANK MERRITT, MD

ENDNOTES

1. Joanna Fantozi, "More Than Half of Americans Skip Breakfast at Least Once a Week, Study Says," *The Daily Meal,* August 18, 2015, http://www.thedailymeal.com/news/healthy-eating/more-half-americans-skip-breakfast-least-once-week-study-says/081815.

2. Dave Asprey, *Head Strong,* 102.

3. Lenna Cooper, "Breakfast Is the Most Important Meal of the Day," *Good Health Magazine*, 1917.

4. Heather Arndt Anderson, *Breakfast: A History* (Lanham, MD: Rowman and Littlefield, 2013), 21-22.

5. Alex Mayyasi, "How Breakfast Became Known as 'The Most Important Meal of the Day,'" *Business Insider,* June 21, 2016, http://www.businessinsider.com/how-breakfast-became-known-as-the-most-important-meal-of-the-day-2016-6?amp.

6. Anderson, *Breakfast: A History,* 23-24.

7. Julie Fink, "The Legend Behind 'The Most Important Meal of the Day,'" *New You,* June 2016, http://www.newyou.com/featured/the-legend-behind-breakfast-is-the-most-important-meal-of-the-day/.

8. "Sugar: The Bitter Truth," *Kolp Institute,* http://kolpinstitute.org/facts-about-sugar/.

9. *New England Journal of Medicine*, 540-548, August 8, 2013.

10. Mark Sisson, "Do You Use Food as a Crutch?" *Mark's Daily Apple,* December 12, 2013, http://www.marksdailyapple.com/do-you-use-food-as-a-crutch/.

11. Catherine and Luke Shanahan, *Deep Nutrition* (New York: Flatiron Books, 2017), 17.

12. Ibid.

13. Ed Silverman, "How Much?! Those New Cholesterol Drugs Could Cost $23 Billion a Year," *Wall Street Journal,* June 9, 2015, https://blogs.wsj.com/pharmalot/2015/06/09/how-much-those-new-cholesterol-drugs-could-cost-23-billion-a-year/; Liz Droge-Young, "Cost of New Cholesterol Drugs Unsustainable, Says Study," *UCSF News Center*, August 16, 2016, https://www.ucsf.edu/news/2016/08/403891/cost-new-cholesterol-drugs-unsustainable-says-study.

14. "More New Cancer Cases Linked to Obesity," *Cancer Treatment Centers of America*, March 10, 2015, http://www.cancercenter.com/discussions/blog/more-new-cancer-cases-linked-to-obesity/.

15. Sam Apple, "An Old Idea, Revived: Starve Cancer to Death," *New York Times,* May 12, 2016, https://www.nytimes.com/2016/05/15/magazine/warburg-effect-an-old-idea-revived-starve-cancer-to-death.html?mcubz=0.

16. "Dom D'Agostino on Disease Prevention, Cancer, and Living Longer," *The Tim Ferriss Podcast,* September 25, 2009, http://tim.blog/2016/09/25/dom-dagostino-on-disease-prevention-cancer-and-living-longer/?utm_source=feedburner&utm_medium=feed&utm_campaign=Feed%3A+timferriss+(The+Blog+of+Author+Tim+Ferriss).

17. Maria Dalamaga et al., "The Role of Adiponectin in Cancer: A Review of Current Evidence," *Endocrine Reviews,* 2012, https://www.ncbi.nlm.nih.gov/pubmed/22547160.

18. "Probiotics Market Size to Exceed USD 64 Billion by 2023: Global Market Insights Inc," *Cision PR Newswire*, May 10, 2016, http://www.prnewswire.com/news-releases/probiotics-market-size-to-exceed-usd-64-billion-by-2023-global-market-insights-inc-578769201.html.

19. A.B. Cruijeiros et al., "Leptin Resistance in Obesity: An Epigenetic Landscape," *Life Sciences,* November 2015, https://www.ncbi.nlm.nih.gov/pubmed/25998029.

20. M.K. Sinha et al., "Evidence of Free and Bound Leptin in Human Circulation: Studies in Lean and Obese Subjects and During Short-Term

Fasting," *Journal of Clinical Investigation,* September 1996, https://www.ncbi.nlm.nih.gov/pmc/articles/PMC507552/.

21. A.A. Gibson et al., "Do Ketogenic Diets Really Suppress Appetite? A Systematic Review and Meta-Analysis," *Obesity Reviews,* January 2015, https://www.ncbi.nlm.nih.gov/pubmed/25402637.

22. Shelly Fan, "The Fat-Fueled Brain: Unnatural or Advantageous?" *Scientific American,* October 1, 2013, https://blogs.scientificamerican.com/mind-guest-blog/the-fat-fueled-brain-unnatural-or-advantageous/.

23. J. Lee et al., "2-Deoxy-D-Glucose Protects Hippocampal Neurons Against Excitotoxic and Oxidative injury: Evidence for the Involvement of Stress Proteins," *Journal of Neuroscience Research,* July 1999, https://www.ncbi.nlm.nih.gov/pubmed/10397635.

24. Dr. Emily Deans, "Your Brain on Ketones," April 2011, https://www.psychologytoday.com/blog/evolutionary-psychiatry/201104/your-brain-ketones.

25. "The Brain's Processing Speed Depends on Myelin," *Life Enhancement,* July 2016.

26. "Routine Periodic Fasting is Good for Your Health, and Your Heart, Study Suggests," *ScienceDaily,* May 20, 2011, www.sciencedaily.com/releases/2011/04/110403090259.htm.

27. A.S. Cornford et al., "Rapid Suppression of Growth Hormone Concentration by Overeating: Potential Mediation by Hyperinsulinemia," *Journal of Clinical Endocrinology & Metabolism,* March 2011, https://www.ncbi.nlm.nih.gov/pubmed/21209037.

28. Interview with Sam George, June 2017.

29. Interview with Randy Rarick, June 2017.

30. Interview with Coach Gene Stallings, July 2017.

31. Interview with Randy Rarick, June 2017.

32. Interview with Peter Furler, June 2017.

33. Interview with Mac Powell, June 2017.

34. Megan Orciari, "Fast Food Companies Still Target Kids with Marketing for Unhealthy Products," *Yale News,* http://news.yale.edu/2013/11/04/fast-food-companies-still-target-kids-

marketing-unhealthy-products; "Snack Food Marketer TV Spend in 2016 Already Tops $100M," *Broadcasting Cable,* http://www.broadcastingcable.com/news/currency/snack-food-marketer-tv-spend-2016-already-tops-100m/154108.

35. Nathan McAlone, "This Chart Shows How More and More Commercials are Being Jammed into NFL Games," *Business Insider,* January 11, 2017, http://www.businessinsider.com/how-many-ads-are-in-nfl-games-chart-2017-1; Aaron Gordon, "The Advertising Football League," *Sports on Earth,* January 30, 2014, http://www.sportsonearth.com/article/67170458/national-football-league-corporate-sponsors-television-ads.

36. Rebecca Lee, "Consumer Reports: What Sleep Remedies Actually Work?" *CBS News,* http://www.cbsnews.com/news/consumer-reports-investigation-sleeping-aids-remedies/.

37. Tim Ferriss, "Dom D'Agostino on Fasting, Ketosis, and the End of Cancer," *The Four Hour Work Week,* http://tim.blog/2015/11/03/dominic-dagostino.

38. Jean-Claude Marquié et al., "Chronic Effects of Shift Work on Cognition: Findings from the VISAT Longitudinal Study," *Journal of Occupational and Environmental Medicine,* 2014, http://oem.bmj.com/content/early/2014/10/08/oemed-2013-101993.short.

39. P.D. Penev, "Association Between Sleep and Morning Testosterone Levels in Older Men," *Sleep,* https://www.ncbi.nlm.nih.gov/pubmed/17520786; E. Van Couter, "Interrelationships Between Growth Hormone and Sleep," *Growth Hormone & IGF Research,* 2000, https://www.ncbi.nlm.nih.gov/pubmed/10984255.

40. Joanna Fantozzi, "More Than Half of Americans Skip Breakfast at Least Once a Week, Study Says," *The Daily Meal,* August 18, 2015, https://www.thedailymeal.com/news/healthy-eating/more-half-americans-skip-breakfast-least-once-week-study-says/081815.

41. Ibid.

42. Interview with Randy Rarick, June 2017.

43. Ibid.

44. "Music Moves Brain to Pay Attention, Stanford Study Finds," *Stanford Medicine,* August 1, 2007, https://med.stanford.edu/news/all-news/2007/07/music-moves-brain-to-pay-attention-stanford-study-finds.html.

45. Adam Pasick, "Better Than Whistling: The Complete Guide to Listening to Music at Work," *Quartz,* March 10, 2014, https://qz.com/185337/the-complete-guide-to-listening-to-music-at-work/.

46. Elizabeth Landau, "This Is Your Brain on Music," *CNN,* February 2, http://www.cnn.com/2013/04/15/health/brain-music-research/.

47. Cory Turner, "This Is Your Brain. This Is Your Brain On Music," *NPR,* September 10, 2014, http://www.npr.org/sections/ed/2014/09/10/343681493/this-is-your-brain-this-is-your-brain-on-music.

48. Interview with Mac Powell, June 2017.

49. Interview with Sam George, June 2017.

50. Interview with Brandon Rager, May 2017.

51. Interview with Coach Gene Stallings, July 2017.

52. Ibid.

53. Caroline E. Jenkinson, Susan Richards et al., "Is Volunteering a Public Health Intervention? A Systematic Review and Meta-Analysis of the Health and Survival of Volunteers," *BMC Public Health,* 2013, https://bmcpublichealth.biomedcentral.com/articles/10.1186/1471-2458-13-773.

54. Interview with Mac Powell, June 2017.

55. Interview with Jesse Billauer, July 2017.

56. Interview with Mac Powell, June 16, 2017.

57. Interview with Randy Rarick, June 2017.

58. "Routine Periodic Fasting Is Good for Your Health and Your Heart, Study Suggests," *ScienceDaily.* May 20, 2011.

59. H. Ding et al., "Fasting Induces a Subcutaneous-to-Visceral Fat Switch Mediated by MicroRNA-149-3p and Suppression of PRDM16," *Nature Communications,* May 2016, https://www.nature.com/articles/ncomms11533.

60. Gretchen Reynolds, "The Best Thing to Eat Before a Workout? Maybe Nothing at All," *New York Times,* April 26, 2017, https://www.nytimes.com/2017/04/26/well/move/the-best-thing-to-eat-before-a-workout-maybe-nothing-at-all.html?mcubz=0.

61. Interview with Brandon Rager, May 2017.

62. Ibid.

63. Mark Mattson, "Why Fasting Bolsters Brain Power: Mark Mattson at TEDx Johns Hopkins University," *TEDx Talks,* 2015, https://www.youtube.com/watch?v=4UkZAwKoCP8.

64. "Episode 7: Mark Mattson Talks About the Benefits of Intermittent Fasting," *STEM-Talk,* April 12, 2016, https://www.ihmc.us/stemtalk/episode007/.

65. Eleanor Maguire, "Cache Cab: Taxi Drivers' Brains Grow to Navigate London's Streets," *Scientific American,* December 2011, https://www.scientificamerican.com/article/london-taxi-memory/.

66. Sandrine Thuret, "You Can Grow New Brain Cells—Here's How," *TED@BCG London,* 2015, https://www.ted.com/talks/sandrine_thuret_you_can_grow_new_brain_cells_here_s_how#t-572127.

67. M. Alirezaei et al., "Short-Term Fasting Induces Profound Neuronal Autophagy," *Autophagy,* August 2010, https://www.ncbi.nlm.nih.gov/pubmed/20534972.

68. Li Liaoliao et al., "Chronic Intermittent Fasting Improves Cognitive Functions and Brain Structures in Mice," *PLos One,* 2013, https://www.ncbi.nlm.nih.gov/pmc/articles/PMC3670843/.

69. Maja Grabacka et al., "Regulation of Ketone Body Metabolism and the Role of PPARα," *International Journal of Molecular Science,* December 2016, https://www.ncbi.nlm.nih.gov/pmc/articles/PMC5187893/.

70. R. Krikorian et al., "Dietary Ketosis Enhances Memory in Mild Cognitive Impairment," *Neurobiology of Aging,* February 2012, https://www.ncbi.nlm.nih.gov/pubmed/21130529.

71. Dr. Bill Lagakos, "Ketosis: Anti-Brain Fog, Neurotransmitters, Dietary Protein, and the Gut Microbiome," *The Poor, Misunderstood Calorie,* October 27, 2013, http://caloriesproper.com/ketosis-anti-brain-fog-neurotransmitters-dietary-protein-and-the-gut-microbiome/.

72. Interview with Randy Rarick, June 2017.

73. Interview with Peter Furler, June 2017.

74. Tom Foxley, Facebook post, July 5, 2017.

75. Interview with Peter Furler, June 2017.

76. Interview with Coach Gene Stallings, July 2017.

77. Ibid.

78. Karen Blumenthal, *Steve Jobs: The Man Who Thought Different,* 265.

Made in the USA
Middletown, DE
21 May 2018